THE
GASTRIC
MIND
BAND®

Published reviews of the first edition of *The Gastric Mind Band*

'This book is the real thing! It helps you understand what you need, not what you want. Great book, great read.' – **Marc**

'The concept is simple, logical and, best of all, it works! I've spent a lifetime (62 years) of clinical obesity and failed diets. Then a book like this comes along and not only understands the mind of an obese person, but has truly come up with a solution. This book has been written by people who actually know what they are talking about.'
– **Mrs St J., Athens**

'I decided to buy this book having battled with weight all of my life. It has only been 10 days, but it has already changed how I think about food and myself.' – **Moomah**

'The book is full of tips and ideas to help the reader to work towards their goals. Anyone with problems relating to weight management should take a look at this book as it is upbeat, positive and can give the reader the motivation to be able to say "yes, I can do this!"'
– **Daphne, Yorkshire, UK**

'I have been on every single diet there is... with limited success and always regaining the weight afterwards. Having read this book, I lost 10 lbs in the first 2 weeks... and that was whilst on holiday. Who loses weight on holiday? What is written in this book is not rocket science... it just makes sense and empowers you to take control.' – **pippinspages**

'This is the most effective and helpful book on weight loss I've ever read. Things like portion control, eating only when hungry and stopping when full are elementary, right? Every diet book addresses these behaviours. If I had ever understood just how to create these behaviours though, my weight would not be an issue.' – **Dixie**

'To call this book the "new bible" is probably an overstatement, but alongside a copy of "the good book" , this book will stay on my bedside table forever! If you have ever dieted in your life or at this moment are overweight, this should be your bedtime reading. You won't be disappointed.' – **Mrs G., Suffolk, UK**

THE
GASTRIC
MIND
BAND®

The Proven, Pain-Free Alternative
to Weight-Loss Surgery

MARTIN AND MARION SHIRRAN
WITH FIONA GRAHAM

HAY
HOUSE

HAY HOUSE
Australia • Canada • Hong Kong • India
South Africa • United Kingdom • United States

First published and distributed in the United Kingdom by:
Hay House UK Ltd, 292B Kensal Road, London W10 5BE
Tel.: (44) 20 8962 1230; Fax: (44) 20 8962 1239.
www.hayhouse.co.uk

Published and distributed in the United States of America by:
Hay House, Inc., PO Box 5100, Carlsbad, CA 92018-5100.
Tel.: (1) 760 431 7695 or (800) 654 5126;
Fax: (1) 760 431 6948 or (800) 650 5115.
www.hayhouse.com

Published and distributed in Australia by:
Hay House Australia Ltd, 18/36 Ralph St, Alexandria NSW 2015.
Tel.: (61) 2 9669 4299; Fax: (61) 2 9669 4144.
www.hayhouse.com.au

Published and distributed in the Republic of South Africa by:
Hay House SA (Pty), Ltd, PO Box 990, Witkoppen 2068.
Tel./Fax: (27) 11 467 8904.
www.hayhouse.co.za

Published and distributed in India by:
Hay House Publishers India, Muskaan Complex, Plot No.3, B-2, Vasant Kunj,
New Delhi – 110 070. Tel.: (91) 11 4176 1620; Fax: (91) 11 4176 1630.
www.hayhouse.co.in

Distributed in Canada by:
Raincoast, 9050 Shaughnessy St, Vancouver, BC V6P 6E5.
Tel.: (1) 604 323 7100; Fax: (1) 604 323 2600

Previously published as *Shirran's Solution: The Gastric Mind Band* (AuthorHouse, 2010)

A catalogue record for this book is available from the British Library.

ISBN: 978-1-78180-053-9

Printed and bound in Great Britain by TJ International Ltd

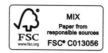

Contents

Acknowledgements

Gastric Mind Band Therapy has been the subject of continual research and development since its launch. This, of course, has only been possible with the help of the literally hundreds of clients who have flown to Spain from various parts of the world to see us. We extend our thanks to all those clients who have allowed us to share their stories.

Of course, each of those clients arrived at our door with their own unique set of issues around food and eating. The extensive knowledge database that we have been able to collect is priceless, and forms the core element of this book, along with the near 6,000 one-to-one clinical hours of therapy time that Marion and I have spent with clients. The result, we believe, is a book based on facts, on real people and on real situations that all readers will be able to relate to.

The support from the media, and their unending coverage of our process, is a constant source of encouragement. It's impossible to name all the publications, but the *Daily Mail*, *Vogue*, *Marie Claire*, *Easy Living* and *Hello!*, along with various TV shows on both sides of the Atlantic are just a small sample of the tremendous exposure we have received.

Our licensee in Cyprus, Dr Theano Kalavana, has been inspirational in the continued development of the process. Gay Jones, our colleague in Pause Button Therapy, has also played a vital role in many areas of improvement.

It is no secret that the book would never have seen the light of day had it not been for the hundreds of hours of hard work and patience of our co-author, Fiona Graham. We hope all those endless hours spent in front of the computer, the sleepless nights and hundreds of miles driven up and down the coast roads of Spain all now seem worthwhile.

Of course, there is very little about weight loss or dieting that has not been covered in one book or another. Marion and I hope that in the pages of *this* book you will discover a new and refreshing approach to obesity, which we believe has now become a very real threat to society. We must thank unreservedly all the people who, unknown to them, we spent many hours observing in restaurants, on flights or just walking down the street doing that thing that we all do – eating!

Finally, we must thank the team at Hay House, especially Carolyn Thorne and our editor, Debra Wolter. This is only our second project with a professional publishing house and we're sure we were sometimes a little naïve. Thanks for your patience.

Martin and Marion Shirran

Foreword

As we all know from print and broadcast media, recent years have seen a dramatic, worldwide rise in obesity. Considered to be one of the most common disorders in medical practice, obesity ranks among the most difficult in terms of management.

After several years of research into the risk factors associated with heart disease, I can quite safely say that obesity is implicated in a number of disorders, including hypertension, Type 2 diabetes mellitus, hyperlipidaemia (elevated levels of lipids in the blood), coronary artery disease, degenerative joint disease and psychological disability.

As most people know from bitter experience, diets will only provide a short-term payoff in the majority of cases. Using conventional dietary methods, just 20 per cent of patients will lose 20lb (9kg) and maintain that loss for over two years. This demonstrates the need to deal with food and hunger in a totally different way. Long-term changes in eating behaviour are essential to maintain weight loss. The team caring for obese individuals can teach useful and effective behavioural techniques.

My friend, Georgina St John, who introduced me to the work of Martin and Marion Shirran, was totally enthused by the couple's commitment and thorough approach. As a clinician, I fully support a method that helps change a patient's relationship with food, and effectively achieves sustainable weight loss. In their therapy, Martin and Marion place great emphasis on choice. You choose to overeat; hence, you may well have to address your emotional urge to eat rather than your physical need, and that is the prime focus of this book.

The Shirrans' method is refreshingly blunt: you wouldn't fill your car to overflowing with fuel, so why do you fill yourself to overflowing with food? We learn to drive on the 'other side of the road' when we go on holiday – isn't it equally important to learn a better eating habit that could save, extend or improve the quality of your life? Many people reading this book will recognize at least some of the anecdotes and embarrassing incidents highlighted, and anyone with a weight problem will relate to them only too well.

Ultimately, it comes down to choice; a choice that can be reversed. This book could save lives – and it might save yours.

Emmanuel Andreadis MD
Dept of Internal Medicine
Evangelismos General Hospital, Athens

About this Book

There's such a wide choice of weight-loss books available today, so why would you believe us rather than other authors? What could *we* possibly know that'll turn your life around more than the other books?

Let's give you an idea. Over the past five years of developing the Gastric Mind Band at our clinic, we've undertaken an enormous amount of research into obesity and weight loss. We've built up nearly 10,000 hours of one-on-one client treatment time, giving us extensive first-hand knowledge of the psychological issues overweight people have around food and eating. Each of our clients arrived with his or her own individual set of problems, and all were desperate to lose their excess weight.

We've helped those clients understand themselves *and* their flawed relationship with food. Each client enabled us to build on our experience and improve our already impressive success rate. We now have a sound understanding of just why people overeat.

So, we know what we're talking about, and we do understand what you'll be thinking. We know where you're coming from, too, and we certainly know exactly where you want to get to. Our knowledge is based on the experiences of real people – young and old, male and female – not faceless statistics.

This is the knowledge and experience we offer you. And with *your* commitment, we *guarantee* success.

The Light-Bulb Moment

How is it possible for an overweight person to be in control of their alcohol consumption, yet always give in when offered a bar of chocolate? How can someone resist trying cocaine all their life, yet regularly succumb to a Big Mac; and how can an ex-smoker turn down the offer of a cigarette, but throw in the towel at the prospect of a chicken korma? These people – and perhaps you, too – show restraint in other areas of their lives, so if they were just able to take that same element of control and apply it to their eating habits, it'd be job done! And all before breakfast!

Our Gastric Mind Band® therapy was developed out of a chance remark and became a phenomenon in a relatively short period of time. In 2007, one of our clients was putting on weight after we'd successfully hypnotized her to stop smoking. In what we now regard as one of the defining moments of our lives, she jokingly asked if we could hypnotize her again, this time to believe that she'd had a gastric band fitted. At the time, we all laughed but, within a few hours, her suggestion had turned from a quip into a light-bulb moment – why had no one thought of this *before*?

That weekend we put together a selection of ideas and therapeutic structures, and two years and much research and development down the line, Martin was 81lb (37kg) lighter, and we had honed that throwaway comment into a well-developed therapy that caught the imagination of members of the medical profession and overweight and obese people around the world.

Nothing could have prepared us for the explosion of worldwide media interest that followed. The work we've done on weight loss – our contribution to solving the global pandemic of obesity – has now featured on TV in Australia, Japan, the Middle East, the USA and across Europe; coverage in print media has been even greater. In the past few years we've opened a clinic with Hazel Newsom in Seattle, USA, with Karen Haggerty in London, and with Dr Theano Kalavana in Cyprus. There are firm plans to add to the network with clinics now opening in Bahrain, Dubai, Abu Dhabi and Denmark.

The extraordinary media interest was matched by a mushrooming of 'copycat' providers, who flooded the market with methods aspiring to emulate our GMB techniques. Having traded for some time, in 2009 we applied for US and EU trademarks. We are confident that, in spite of claims by other 'virtual banding' services, we are the originators of the method, and with our dedication to ongoing research and development, the Elite Clinics network will remain the premier providers.

Our Pause Button Therapy® (PBT) – a key element of the GMB therapy – has been developed into a technique in its own right. Now the subject of a book (*Pause Button Therapy*, Hay House, 2012), it was presented at the 1st International Conference on Time Perspective and to university students and other delegates globally.

The therapy provided to GMB clients at our Elite Clinics in Spain, and in other licensed GMB clinics around the world, has developed a great deal since we started; the success rate is also continuing to improve. We are keen to become partners in academic research on weight loss, and have built up a considerable amount of data for future analysis. Dr Theano Kalavana is carrying out hospital-based research in Cyprus, and we are exploring sources of funding for MRI scan research of clients' brain patterns whilst undergoing GMB treatment.

Your GMB Journey

In this book you'll be taken on a journey of self-discovery, learning about your psychological relationship with food. In the same way as if you were a client sitting in our clinic, we'll help you to see how you make the wrong food choices; the times when you eat for the wrong reasons; the many different triggers that you have which have led you down the road towards obesity. Moreover, we'll give you the tools to make major lifestyle changes, and introduce you to the 'Diet Terrorists' and the chaos they cause those trying to take control of their weight.

As you read the book, you'll meet our better-known success stories: Sarah Jayne Hart, from Wales, who shed half her body weight and is still at her target weight three years after starting with GMB, and Kay Lindley, whose diabetes now requires minimal intervention as a result of her weight loss. Other less well-known – but equally happy – clients provide testimonials.

We guarantee that you'll recognize most of the things they say as they describe how they thought they'd never get to grips with eating normally. They felt they could never succeed where they'd always failed in the past – putting back on all the weight they'd lost. But their experiences with GMB will show you that it's possible to get the weight off, keep it off, and achieve your long-term goals. And, what's more, that you shouldn't diet at all!

You'll also read about a client who came to the clinic for help after experiencing a catastrophic surgical gastric band failure that resulted in her almost losing her life, and, then having recovered, fearing she'd always be overweight. Surgery was not the miracle cure she'd anticipated!

This book provides the reader with the closest thing possible to a course of GMB therapy in our clinic − it covers every component, including the hypnotherapy and visualization. We talk frankly about your eating habits, and we illustrate how no overweight person should carry on the way they are without being brought face to face with the appalling health risks attached to being overweight.

We'll ask you whether your reason for wanting to shed excess weight is to fit into a bikini next summer, or to avoid losing a limb to Type 2 diabetes. Whether you can see the irony of driving a car with a seat belt and an airbag to protect you in case of an accident, and at the same time eating a bar of chocolate that will guarantee you carry excess weight which is statistically far more likely to kill you. In the UK, around 1,850 people a year die in road traffic accidents, yet some 30,000 die from obesity-related conditions.[1,2]

You'll be asked questions about your food choices, and about your relationship with meals and eating − not only today, but when you were younger, too. About the triggers that you − and all overweight people − have that lead you to overeat. About the effects your weight problem has on you, and on your family and friends. About how you might feel, and what your life would be like, a year from now, if you were slim. Soon, you'll realize you're at a fork in the road of your life. A place where the choice of direction is entirely up to you. And, finally, you'll see just how few changes you need to make in order to set off along a totally different pathway to the fat, bloated and unhappy one you're on now.

Most importantly, you'll realize this *is* possible. You *can be* that slimmer, fitter, healthier person next year − if you have the motivation. We are passionate about our therapy, and we pull no punches: we make it quite clear, in the clinic and in the pages of this book, that you won't achieve a thing until you're completely ready, sure of your motivation, and, above all, totally committed. You have to believe *you can do this*, and the evidence from our past clients and readers says that you can.

You can't live without food, so it's vital that you learn to live with it. This is the start of the rest of your life. Right here. Right now.

We are emphatic in our belief that, if you are totally committed, you will achieve the weight loss you desire with the Gastric Mind Band therapy. However, anyone undertaking any weight-loss programme is advised to discuss their proposed actions with their GP.

And, as is done with people seeking gastric band surgery, at the Elite Clinics we ensure we are confident that clients are not suffering from eating disorders such as anorexia or bulimia before proceeding with treatment.

'It's brilliant. I don't feel like I'm on a diet. I can eat whatever I choose – it's just making the right choices.'
SARAH JAYNE HART, GMB CLIENT: WEIGHT LOSS 144LB (65KG), 2009–2011

Glossary of Therapies

You will see references to several therapies throughout the book.

CBT (Cognitive Behaviour Therapy) asks the individual to consider that their thoughts can be inaccurate – they are *thoughts* as opposed to *logical, rational facts*. Once they recognize these 'sabotaging thoughts' they can begin to overcome them.

NLP (Neuro-Linguistic Programming) enables people to change their experience of reality by altering how they represent it to themselves. By understanding and working with the ways that language affects the subconscious, and techniques that reorganize the underlying sensory data in the mind, NLP empowers people to make the changes they desire. It incorporates creative visualization and enables the widening of beliefs so you can 'see' yourself in a different, better state of mind – with all the changes that accompany your new self-image. Focusing on this new 'blueprint' enables your subconscious mind to create a new set of responses and behaviours.

Guided Imagery is a technique similar to NLP in which the client is encouraged to see into the future by being taken through alternative scenarios in their mind's eye.

Hypnotherapy works because any suggestions made while the subconscious mind is receptive during deep relaxation are far more likely to be 'accepted'; the subconscious mind is more influential on our behaviour than the conscious mind, so in day-to-day life the suggestions can begin to take effect without any conscious effort.

Life Architecture is the name we've given to a therapy we've developed that is a combination of various therapies, each of which is used to underpin the other.

Pause Button Therapy® is our easy-to-learn method of adopting the function buttons of a remote control device to allow people to freeze time and fast-forward to see the consequences of their actions.

The Elite Clinics

You'll also see references to Elite Clinics. This is the clinic in Spain owned and operated by us, Martin and Marion Shirran, as the founders of GMB and PBT. We offer a range of therapies at the clinic.

While we have striven to make this book as comprehensive as possible, it can never replace the considerable benefits obtained by sitting on a one-to-one basis with a therapist. For details of GMB clinics and the locations and availability of sessions, see page 271 or visit www.gmband.com

Finally, we have spoken to a number of GMB clients for case study material and, where appropriate, names and details have been changed to preserve anonymity.

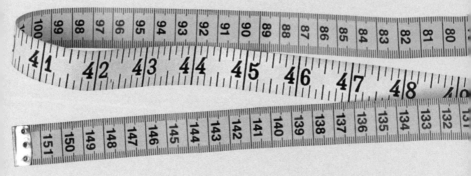

PART 1

THE BACKGROUND TO GMB

Chapter 1
Obese? Moi?

Obese. Obesity. Martin hates these words with a passion.

'I can remember lying in a hospital bed after being admitted to have my appendix removed,' he recalls. 'The surgeon came to see me before the operation with four trainee doctors. He was talking to them about me, my condition and the surgery, but he spoke about me as if I wasn't there. I was described simply as an "obese male".

'More than 25 years later, I remember those words vividly. I do recall that, at the time, I thought I was a little overweight, but in that moment I was labelled as clinically obese. That wasn't pleasant at all.'

Martin's experience is not unusual these days, though. No one is just 'chubby' any more; people don't have a 'spare tyre'; kids no longer have 'puppy fat'. More often than not they're now labelled as 'obese' – which is, as Martin says, a truly horrible word.

Of course, the problem of global obesity is no less real because Martin doesn't like the word. Some experts believe that obesity is a bigger threat to the planet than global warming.[1] However, as a word – as the effect it has on people – obesity is like that other dreaded word; the one that's even more frightening, the one guaranteed to bring you out in a cold sweat. We're talking about cancer.

These days, no one has a 'lump', nor do they have a 'growth' or a 'tumour' – it's cancer. Just mentioning the word sends people into shock; we imagine that the very sound of it must send a possible sufferer's immune system into near total shutdown – just at a time when they surely need their defences to be working at maximum efficiency.

Martin once had a partner who found a lump in her breast. The doctor thought it was a cyst – which, statistically, they usually are – and over a few weeks, as expected, it disappeared. A year or so later, a lump came up under her arm. It was never discussed as cancer in the lymph nodes, just as a cyst. We do wonder whether the word cancer is bandied about a little too freely today. Would it not be beneficial to keep the patient positive? At least until they receive a full diagnosis.

We mention all of this because, in a similar vein, when clients come to the clinic we always strive to ensure they are never overwhelmed by the problem of being overweight. We want them to be, and remain, 100 per cent positive. A person's absolute belief and positivity in their ability to succeed is paramount in all change scenarios in their life, not least in the area of weight loss.

We are adamant that it's essential for our clients to continue believing that this situation, this problem they have with excess weight, can always be reversed. Sure, we use the words obese and obesity, but reluctantly, and only when and where it's appropriate.

So, rather than saying: 'Well, you're overweight, maybe even obese. You need to lose five stone (31kg) and that'll take at least eight months', we phrase it differently. We'll say: 'Sure, you have a weight problem, but you know, you needn't worry because we often see clients with far more weight to lose than you do. You can, with a little help and certainly no pain, fix it – not just temporarily but permanently. We're here to help you and show you how – right here, right now. That's if you're ready, of course!'

The same applies to you as you begin to read this book. As you start putting our therapy into action, positivity is vital. You *can* shift that excess weight. You *can* be healthier and fitter, and look and feel better. The Gastric Mind Band is here to help you, and you *will* be able to do it. Starting now.

The GMB therapy we've developed will take you into the eye of the dieting storm, offering you an exciting new approach and introducing you to issues you'd never considered were connected to your overeating problems. It puts a spotlight on your complex emotional relationship with food and shows you how to rethink the whole issue of being overweight. In the pages of this book, we hope you will, maybe for the first time in your life, have the tools and the knowledge to finally take control.

Why Do You Want to Shift Your Excess Weight?

Okay, let's be frank. Most of the readers of this book are probably overweight to some degree or another, and each will have his or her reasons for wanting to reverse the situation, whether health or vanity related.

Your reasons for wanting to lose weight may not be the same as your neighbour's, or his father's, or his teenage niece's – everyone's reasons are different. It's often down to appearance, or wanting to wear nicer/different clothes, or to look better for a partner.

It's a surprising fact that most overweight people rarely consider the amount of damage they're doing to their bodies by keeping them so unhealthily fat. Their thoughts are stuck in today – in eating *now* – not in what'll happen next year, or how unfit or ill they might be 10 years from now. Hopefully, you will be starting to understand that, in the same way as in all other aspects of your life, with weight you need to accept the very important consequences of your actions.

You may not be super morbidly obese; maybe you just know you need to lose weight before it affects your health any further. *You* know it, *we* know it, and most of all, you want rid of the very idea of it. But, do you know what you're doing to yourself? Let's hope you do – or maybe let's hope you don't, or you'd have changed your eating habits a long time ago.

Before you start on the road to a new you, it's important to lay bare the gravity of the problem. You may be familiar with some of what we're about to say, but it might help you to focus your thoughts, and establish the right mindset prior to starting out on this very important journey.

Do You Have a Fear of Death?

This is such a powerful question. Stop for a moment and ask yourself, 'Are you scared of dying?' Many overweight people carry on blindly, unaware of what their excess fat could be doing to the quality of their life ahead. In short, how it could affect their life expectancy. How do *you* feel about the possibility of a shorter life, or chronic illness, or death?

Of course, many people lead unhealthy lives and still survive to a ripe old age, but the trend is going the other way. Tens of thousands of deaths in the USA alone are caused as a direct result of obesity.[2] Worldwide, obesity has more than doubled since 1980;[3] and by 2008, some 1.5 billion adults over the age of 20 were overweight.[4]

The UK government says that in 2010/11, there were 11,574 hospital admissions caused directly by obesity – that's 10 times greater than in 2000/01.[5] It also says that more than 20 million British people are now considered overweight or obese.[6] As long ago as 2007, it was calculated that rising obesity would add £5.5 billion to the UK's NHS bill by 2050.[7]

In 2010, more than a million weight-loss prescriptions were dispensed in the UK. This was actually a slight drop from 2009, possibly because two of the three main obesity drugs had been withdrawn.[8] But, of course, pills only treat the symptoms, they'll never fix the cause.

Today, obesity contributes to as much as 20 per cent of all cancer-related deaths,[9] yet until 50 years ago, obesity was so uncommon that it wasn't considered important enough to keep records of it.[10]

There are many, many health downsides to being overweight. We can't possibly cover them all, but here's a brief overview of just four of them. It doesn't make comfortable reading, but it's something that every overweight person, whatever their age, should take a close look at – however much they may not want to. It may be a good idea to create your own list showing the diseases and conditions you fear the most.

Don't dig your grave with your own knife and fork.
ENGLISH PROVERB

Type 2 Diabetes

This disease is reckoned to be among the top five killers in most developed countries. More than 75 per cent of people with Type 2 diabetes – some statistics suggest that it's as much as 85 per cent in the USA – are overweight.[11] The high blood glucose levels associated with diabetes increase the risk of heart disease, stroke, high blood pressure, kidney failure, and poor circulation, which can lead to limb amputation.

Damage to the retina of the eye is another common problem associated with diabetes, and it can lead to blindness. Globally, the number of diabetes sufferers is predicted to top 550 million by 2030,[12] and in the UK, the cost of treating the disease is projected to rise to £16.9bn ($27bn) by 2035, threatening to 'bankrupt' the NHS.[13]

Stroke

This condition is the third largest killer in the UK, and the NHS spends £2.3 billion a year on treating stroke victims.[14] A stroke is usually caused by a blockage or rupture of a blood vessel in the brain, and can leave the victim paralysed down one side of their body. It can also affect their speech and vision, among other things. Obesity is a high indicator of the likelihood of suffering a stroke.

Cancer

Every year in the UK, some 13,000 people could avoid getting cancer if they were a healthy weight. The World Health Organization (WHO) says that, after tobacco, obesity/overweight are the most important known avoidable causes of cancer. Obesity could be linked to the doubling of kidney cancer rates over the past 35 years.[15] Other types of cancer known to be linked to weight are colon, breast, uterus, rectal, pancreas, prostate, gallbladder, and thyroid cancers.[16]

Heart Disease

One fifth of all heart disease cases in the UK can be attributed to obesity, and heart disease can lead to heart attacks and angina. A heart attack is caused by a blockage or rupture of one of the main blood vessels around the heart, and is usually extremely painful. Even after ruling out other risk factors, such as high blood pressure and diabetes, obese men have a 60 per cent greater risk of suffering a fatal heart attack than non-obese men.[17]

This is just a snapshot of the better-known health risks of obesity. If you need any further convincing, there's a more extensive – though still not exhaustive – summary in Chapter 11. Maybe you should read and digest this information – it could increase your level of motivation for change.

> *'When it comes to eating right and exercising, there is no "I'll start tomorrow." Tomorrow is disease.'*
> **V.L. ALLINEARE**

A Weapon Against Obesity

Now that you've read the brief overview of Type 2 diabetes, stroke, cancer and heart disease, it's possible that you have a different focus to your reasons for wanting to shed some excess weight. Whatever your personal goals or motives, though, we believe that GMB is an exciting new tool – not only in your personal battle with your weight but also in the global battle against obesity.

The fact that there's been extraordinary press coverage for our therapy is great for us personally and professionally, but the stories in the media focused, rather predictably, on GMB's 'hook' – the seemingly magical effect of the Gastric Mind Band hypnotherapy session. Little, if any, mention has been made of the rest of the therapy; you could be forgiven for thinking that our whole approach is very 'lightweight', in more ways than one.

However, there's much, much more to GMB than just the one 'banding' session. There are the many thought-provoking questions, answers, research, challenges, suggestions, techniques and lessons in the therapy. There's our unique Pause Button Therapy®, which helps you 'freeze' time – giving you the thinking space you might need to avoid making the wrong food choices. PBT is key to GMB, and *no other virtual banding system can offer it.*

We are completely serious and committed to the ongoing development of the therapy, and we really hope the opportunity will arise to bring GMB to a wider audience through health organizations and professionals, both in the UK and internationally.

Being overweight or obese is a symptom of overeating; of having an unhealthy relationship with food. The GMB therapy aims to deal with the symptom and, more importantly, to treat the *cause* of the problem. That's how you get permanent results.

'I've come to understand that for years I'd thought being overweight was for one reason, when in fact it became quite clear it was another, completely different thing! I feel so positive; I really think this is going to work for me.'
GMB CLIENT **S.K.**

The Bigger Picture

Being overweight is primarily the result of overeating. Overeating happens for numerous reasons, many of which are anchored in the past. Perhaps some emotional event caused you to begin eating for security, comfort or protection. The memory of the event remains sealed in your subconscious mind, even if you've forgotten it consciously.

This could be as simple as the fact that, when you were a child, your parents told you to eat up everything on your plate, perhaps adding for good measure that well-worn phrase, 'think of all the starving children in Africa!' Sayings like this follow us into adulthood, even though the logic behind this one is rather strange – how can the fact that we are overeating possibly compensate for the poor undernourished children in Africa?

Add the stresses and strains of daily life to the overeating – and the fact that we move our bodies around far less than ever before – and the result is an obesity problem that's spiralling out of control. While we yearn for the body beautiful – or at least the body socially acceptable – diet companies promise quick fixes, miracle solutions, shakes, pills, and all manner of new-fangled machines, each promising something we hope we can achieve by taking short cuts.

It's not rocket science: we know that we need to lose weight and improve our health. But we must wise up to the fact that we need to change the reasons, and the ways, we eat and move. And, hopefully, get away from the idea of 'dieting' – on their own, diets rarely produce permanent results, because they don't address the important, complex and sometimes highly emotional relationship that exists between overweight people and food.

'I've been on and off diets since I was 14; all of them worked, and all of them failed. So, in my mid-50s and fat, GMB sounded too good to be true… my husband thought I was mad, but I knew that if I didn't do something my health would start to suffer. Now my motivation is great, and the weight is coming off slowly and steadily. I don't mind how long it takes – I know that this time I'll get there.'
GMB client W.N.

Most 'diets' cannot be sustained for more than a short period of time because they are restrictive – the diet becomes a form of self-torture that you endure temporarily, going against all your usual eating habits while being deprived of many of your favourite foods. Deprivation simply creates stronger desire, so if you are following a diet that creates 'forbidden' foods, you end up craving all the foods you are not 'allowed' to have.

When you finish 'dieting' you revert to your 'normal' eating habits, which in fact means overeating, and eating for the wrong reasons. You also tend to reward yourself with all the things that you have been craving so much during the diet, and as a result, all the weight, if not even more, goes back on again. Because dieting doesn't address the underlying psychological craving for excess food, an overweight person ends up on a seemingly permanent roller-coaster ride of yo-yo dieting, losing their self-confidence along the way and feeling more and more despondent about their continuous battle with their weight.

In this book we're going to help *you* put an end to this all-too-familiar pattern once and for all. We'll help you to create a better relationship with food – one that you'll be able to maintain for the rest of your life.

Will You Spare Us a Week or Two?

The way to look at *long-term* weight loss – a permanent change in your eating habits – is to see it as 'chunking'. This means looking at each little success as valuable in its own right. If you have 6 stone (38kg) to lose, you won't be able to shift it in a fortnight. It could take you 42 weeks – 10 months or so – probably a bit longer.

You can see chunking as enjoying the *journey* to your destination as much as the *destination* itself. You can enjoy the whole experience – booking the journey, packing the cases, getting to the airport, boarding the plane… Do it a bit at a time.

It's only too easy to feel that there's *so* much weight to shift, and that it's all going to take *such* a long time. But, never forget that today is the last time you'll feel this bad about your weight. In a fortnight's time you'll feel better. You might not yet be slim, but you'll still feel better. You'll be feeling more positive, and slightly more comfortable in your clothes. And certainly not as bad as you did two weeks earlier. It's a gradual change – not only in the shape of your body, but in how you feel about yourself.

Someone with 5 stone (31.8kg) to lose would probably take the best part of a year to shift it, and all they can see is getting to a size 12. We'd say to them: 'Where in the world do you really want to go?' They might opt for Los Angeles, so we'd then say: 'See it as a 12-month world cruise, taking in some wonderful places – Portugal, Barbados, Curacao, Panama, Guatemala – and you're going to enjoy all of them on the way to LA. It'll be brilliant when you get there, but the journey will be wonderful, too.'

If you're 15st 11lb (100.5kg) and want to be 9st 7lb (60.5kg), you can enjoy being 15st (95.5kg). It's wonderful compared to your original weight, isn't it? Treat yourself and look forward to the next stop on the cruise – which may be 14st 7lb

(92.3kg), or 14st 2lb (90kg). Enjoy that, and then do the next bit. Don't say, 'I'm not going to relax, and I'm not going to reward myself until I get to my target weight.' Visualize it as a long-term project, because at some point your weight will plateau.

'I'm aiming to be one pound (0.45kg) lighter at the end of the week' sounds so much easier than 'I need to drop 6st 9lb (42kg) over the next eight months'.

WHAT YOU'VE LEARNED IN THIS CHAPTER

- To forget about dieting – it doesn't help!

- Our face-to-face, in-clinic therapy is a winning formula – and you've got most of it in your hands right now!

- Stroke, heart disease, heart attacks, diabetes, cancer... the list of conditions related to being overweight goes on and on.

- Think about this, and then turn the page and start doing something about it.

Chapter 2

Giraffes, Sparrows and Obesity

So, what are *your* reasons for wanting to shed your excess weight? Do they include a desire to impress your partner? Improve your physical appearance? Increase your energy levels? Follow fashion trends? Or might they be the very real risk of developing coronary heart disease, Type 2 diabetes, colon cancer, or one of the many other obesity-related conditions and diseases? This question is for you to consider – we'll be asking it again later! For the moment, though, here's another simple question: 'Why do people eat?'

Do we eat dinner because we're hungry, or because the clock tells us it's 7 p.m? Do we stop eating because we're full, or because our plate's empty? It's almost certainly the latter, so there's no actual physical connection with the body's needs. Has it become a custom in your home to eat at 7 p.m? Or a social event? When you're alone, why do you have dinner? What's the reason? Is it just because it's 7 p.m., or is there another reason?

If you travel through a time zone and arrive at your destination when you 'should' be asleep but everyone's about to have lunch, what do you do? If you eat, ask yourself why.

> **Sad people eat when they're not really hungry; happy people watch a good film, listen to music, write a letter or an email, take a walk, or enjoy a long hot soak in a bubble bath. They wake each morning feeling refreshed, not fat and sad.**

Ask yourself if you even *know* what it is to be hungry. Maybe we're all stuffing food in our mouths so quickly that our brains never get a chance to think, 'Hey, wait, I'm not hungry', let alone, 'Stop, I'm full!' Would anyone in the Western world recognize a true hunger pang any more? Has anyone even *experienced* one in the past 10 years?

One pound of fat (0.45kg) contains 3,500 calories. So you only have to be eating 135 calories a day more than your body needs to be putting on one stone (6.3kg) a year. 135 calories is not a mega meal, either − it's less than the number of calories in a standard-sized Snickers bar, or a small glass of wine, and it's less than a quarter of a Big Mac. It's really only one large apple a day more than your body needs before you've piled on a stone (6.3kg) a year. If you've put on weight faster than that, you've been eating much more than your body needs − and it's showing in the most obvious (and visible) way − on the scales.

But the good news is that it's quite easy to skip those extra 135 calories a day. Just don't eat that bar of chocolate; or have a glass of water instead of that wine. Small daily steps like this add up to massive results, because you're reducing your intake in the same way as eating when you *weren't* hungry added up to those rolls of fat.

You need to understand the thought processes that lead you to eat (and overeat). Understand that just thinking – and eating – in the here and now won't achieve your goal. That piece of chocolate cake may look good, but the taste will last perhaps two minutes. Is it *really* worth it, just for two minutes?

However, if you do eat the chocolate cake, it isn't the end of the world. Get back on the bike, and learn that it was just a lapse. Make sure that it never happens again, but take knowledge from it. Learn *why* you picked up the cake. Where were you? Who were you with? Any lapse, any mistake, is not *such* a bad thing, and it's a great way of learning how *not* to do it again.

***Eating a piece of chocolate cake is a lapse
and nothing else – it's a single event, a one-off.
A relapse is reverting to filling your face with
cake day in, day out, and not bothering to
'get back on the bike' again.***

Building a New Relationship with Food

Improving your relationship with food is vital to the process of shedding excess weight because, try as you might have done in the past, you can't avoid food. You need to eat in order to live. You have to face food choices several times a day, so it's essential to retrain yourself to understand *how and why* you made the wrong choices before, and to learn new, healthier habits for the future. We will teach you how to recognize your triggers; how to stop and identify the first thought that leads to you making bad food choices.

When you experience that first thought – and you're within moments of reaching for food when you really don't need to eat – it's the perfect time to use your 'Pause Button'. We'll explain more about that later in the book, but whenever you find yourself in these seemingly hopeless situations, all you need to do is imagine that you have a remote control for your life (similar to the one you use to operate your TV/DVD player) so you can pause/fast-forward/rewind as and when necessary to see ahead to the consequences of your actions and avoid making the wrong food choices.

You didn't put your excess weight on all at once, so you can't expect to lose it all overnight. Of course you can have a target, a goal, but it's important to enjoy all the smaller steps along the way, too.

Tell yourself that you're going to lose one pound (0.45kg) this week,** not **that you need to lose four stone (25kg) before that wedding next Easter.

If you've lost 4lb (1.8kg) yet still have 4st 12lb (31kg) to go, celebrate the fact that you now weigh that much less than you did a fortnight ago. The same applies to the next few pounds, or even the next half a pound (0.22kg): be positive rather than thinking about how much more you want to lose and feeling negative. Being positive has a knock-on effect on how you make choices.

Some of the factors that influence your food choices – which, presumably, have been seriously flawed up until now – include:

- Personal triggers. We'll be looking at whether you're driven to eat by the smell wafting out from a baker's shop, or an argument, or boredom.

- Want, need, desire and craving. We'll be exploring the differences between these.

- Seemingly Irrelevant Decisions.[1] An example of this is when you go to a party you're ambivalent about because you know there'll be a hearty buffet to tuck into.

- Here and Now Thinking. This is when you only see the next few seconds in front of you – to the pork pie or the ice cream. You know those things are going to be really yummy – and that they're what you need right here and now – but you're not looking at the medium- or long-term consequences of what you're doing.

- The Diet Terrorists. We'll explain who these are, and how they create chaos in the minds of dieters the world over.

- Low Frustration Tolerance (LFT).[2] We'll show you how this concept can help you tolerate hunger, and stop you from being frightened of it.

Recognizing these factors/triggers means you can avoid reacting in the wrong way and reaching for the doughnuts, bar of chocolate, or whatever. You can get on top of them, but you need the tools, and as you work through the book, you'll get them.

THE LAST SUPPER

For some reason, most overweight people seem to have a problem when eating out. They manage to eat carefully for weeks while at home, but as soon as they walk through the door of a restaurant, they crash and burn. Along with their endless list of excuses for the collapse of their healthy eating regime, this is often down to what we call 'The Last Supper' syndrome.

Overweight people often seem to treat a visit to a restaurant as if it were their last ever meal. They must have it all, and have it tonight! They feel compelled to order their favourite starter as well as a main course, and the house special dessert too. It's as if they feel this is their last chance; they cannot say no to anything, least of all the dessert. They treat it as 'The Last Supper'. Next time you're in a restaurant, take a look around and you'll see the phenomenon for yourself!

Your GMB Toolbox

Gaining an understanding of this flawed way of thinking, and more, amounts to you being given a great big toolbox and a hard hat: the toolbox to understand how to change your attitudes towards food, and the hard hat to protect yourself against your own flawed thinking – and against those dangerous 'terrorists' who are out to foil your best intentions.

There are so many elements to consider when taking a closer look at your dodgy food choices. You have to pick out those that apply to you, and learn how to stop yourself and 'freeze time' before every meal to see if you *really* need to eat what you've chosen. You've probably never done that before! We'll show you how your mind ambushes you, and how to control it.

In GMB we mix approaches, and underpin one therapy with another: it's what we call 'Life Architecture'. We merge 'science-based' therapies such as CBT with NLP and Guided Imagery, plus, of course, Pause Button Therapy (PBT). All these methods appear throughout the book – sometimes several times – but in different ways.

You – and no one else – need to design a plan for living and enjoying your life tailored to your own individual needs, fears, dreams and aspirations. It won't contain any forbidden foods and nothing is banned; there are no themes, daily calorie-counting, fat points, none of it. Just a normal relationship with something you have to face daily just to stay alive.

What's with the Giraffes?

It's simple! Giraffes, sparrows, squirrels – and virtually any other wild animal you care to name – eat when they're hungry, until they're satisfied, and then they stop eating. Have you ever seen a fat sparrow? Do they eat the seed off the ground until it's all gone and they can't fly away? No, they eat what they need and then leave. Would a giraffe pull off and then eat so many leaves from a tree that it couldn't walk? Not a chance! Squirrels, too. They'll go out and collect lots of nuts for food. But do they then eat them all until they're fat? No – they eat what they need, and then bury the rest for when they're hungry again. Obesity is almost exclusively a disease that affects the human species. The squirrel says, 'that's enough: bury'. Squirrels have got it sussed!

It's a similar story with disease. It's likely that we can all name someone who died of cancer, or a heart attack, or liver disease. But how many animals die each year from obesity-related conditions? How many of those are captive or domesticated, and how many are wild? Think about what that might mean.

And what do we humans do? We sit there and eat – one, maybe two, courses, and then order pudding. No one orders pudding because they're *hungry*, do they? How can they be? They've just had two courses, probably a glass of wine, and a bread roll, too. So we've had three or more courses, and then we go on to eat between these meals as well. We eat and eat, even though we're not actually hungry. How stupid are we?

If you've been on diets before and they've failed, it'll be because a diet doesn't address what's going on inside your head. A diet never addresses the whole concept of emotional eating – that is, eating when you're bored or stressed or angry. It's our belief that diets can't work in the long term because you always 'go back' to your old ways unless you've changed your thinking. GMB is about giving you the defence mechanisms you need. You've got to be able to enjoy yourself and live – and eat – in the real world.

There are plenty of people who've lost a considerable amount of weight with different slimming groups, or diet systems, and then put it all back on because none of them ever get to the subconscious part of the decision-making process. They address the symptom, but not the cause.

MORE IMPORTANT THINGS TO DO THAN EAT

A friend of ours called Gary travels down from the town of Northampton, in England's East Midlands, to Gatwick, near London, four days a week, and one day he visited us for a coffee. He wasn't usually so blunt, but he asked if we could make him a couple of pieces of toast with his drink.

He told us that on his way to work the previous day, there'd been an accident and a traffic jam, and the journey had taken nearly four hours. He was then in meetings all day and didn't have time for a lunch break. After work, he had a stopover at Heathrow to collect his son, where he found the flight was delayed. He finally got home at 10 p.m., but then had to sort through 40 emails. After doing that, he fell asleep on the sofa, where he awoke the next day before heading off to another meeting. He arrived at our home not feeling too good and realized he'd forgotten to eat the previous day.

In nearly two days, all Gary had consumed was one coffee. This was only because he was so busy; so much was going on, and, of course, because food was not the most important thing in his life. He was quite happy – pleased he was slim and healthy, and that his life was so full. All he needed was to have something to eat and be off again.

What's Your Motivation?

Where weight loss is concerned, motivation is as important as what you eat. It's also as important as restricting calories, yet it gets talked about nowhere near enough. Whether you've chosen Weight Watchers, Cambridge, Hay, Scarsdale, whatever, motivation is key.

Imagine your doctor said to you: 'You've got Type 2 diabetes. Your toes are already looking a little bit grey, so you're probably looking at amputation unless you do something about your weight.' Would that be enough to motivate you? Would your motivation be so high that you wouldn't need us? If you enjoyed a 100 per cent recovery after a mild stroke, and the doctor said you'd been lucky this time, but that the next one could leave you paralysed, would you be able to lose weight?

If someone said they'd pay you £500,000 to lose all your excess weight, would you sign up for it and succeed? That's motivation! So why haven't you been motivated to lose weight before? Maybe there's a discrepancy between what you *think* you want to do and what you're *actually* doing.

We'll teach you to understand your motivation, but at the end of the day it's down to you whether it's important enough to you to make the changes.

Our minds have a great influence on our behaviour, and the mind works best when it concentrates on a positive goal. We tend to talk about 'losing' weight, but our minds think that if we lose something we can't rest until we find it again. A much more positive concept for your mind to accept is for you to see yourself as not *losing* weight, but *getting rid of* excess, unwanted fat, and moving closer to your target weight as a result. We will actively strive to get rid of rubbish and things we don't want in our lives any more.

Although 99 per cent of diets *should* succeed, nowhere near that many are successful in the long term. The average 45-year-old British woman has tried 61 diets, and will spend 31 years doing so.[3] And more than 20 per cent of British women are on a permanent diet.[4] Yet many do all this and lose *no weight* in the long term.

Virtually all weight-loss programmes can be successful if you stick to them. But why don't people stick to them? Because they're not sufficiently motivated, and they don't understand what's really going on. You have to ask yourself two questions: 'Why am I doing this?' and 'Why do I want to lose weight?', and answer truthfully to get close to discovering the solution.

The problem with eating is seldom down to the food or the stomach. It's psychological. You're eating for some reason other than hunger: because you're bored; because it's 7 p.m; because you're lonely; because you've found some leftovers in the fridge. The word 'hunger' seldom slips in.

When you tuck into that chocolate cake, or decide to have dinner, is it because you're hungry? Where do you feel the hunger? In your brain? Your throat? Your stomach? In the split-second decision to eat, the one question rarely asked is, 'Am I hungry?'

As long as whatever you want to accomplish is realistic, achievable and important enough to you, there's no reason why you can't make it happen – the only thing stopping you is yourself!

Hunger, Craving and Desire

You have to understand the difference between these states; it's fundamental to understanding our approach to food.

Medical research says that hunger has nothing to do with the stomach. It seems that people who've had their stomach removed still get hungry. We're told that the part of the brain involved in hunger is the lateral hypothalamus.[5] Your brain can detect when your blood falls short of certain nutrients – amino acids, carbohydrates, proteins – and sends the message that you're hungry and are ready to eat. And when you're hungry, you'll eat anything. If you say, 'I'm absolutely starving, I've got to have a fillet steak,' don't kid yourself, because those two things can't go together. If you're *really* hungry, an apple, a piece of toast or some plain grilled fish will do. If you want a fillet steak, that's a *craving*.

Are you hungry 30 minutes after eating? Really? How about three hours? A day? A week? The human body can survive for up to 40 days without food, providing water is taken,[6] so you can't possibly be truly starving after a few hours!

If you eat a bag of crisps, it won't satisfy your body's needs, so an hour later your brain will say, 'I'm still hungry, give me more'.[7] This cycle of eating junk but never fulfilling what your body needs nutritionally is the cycle of obesity, because people are just eating – thinking that stuffing junk food in their mouths, anything that's available, anything they fancy at the time, is going to take the hunger away. It doesn't.

Something you may not know is that the first sign of dehydration is hunger, not thirst.[8] So what do you do? You sit there, dying of thirst and say, 'I'm hungry', and eat a cheese roll. Five minutes later, though, you'll be 'hungry' again because it wasn't food you needed, it was water… so you'll eat another cheese roll. And be 'hungry' again in five minutes. You'll be getting fatter and fatter instead of just having a drink of water.

If you think you're hungry, try having a glass of water. If you're still hungry 15 or 20 minutes later, then eat. If you're not hungry, it was simply that you were thirsty!

The next time you reach for something to eat, stop before you put it in your mouth and ask yourself, 'Am I hungry?' If the answer is no, what emotion or feeling are you experiencing that's prompting you to eat?

A newborn baby knows it wants milk. It doesn't know its BMI or height-to-weight ratio, it just drinks, knows it's not hungry any more and then stops. And that's how simple it has to be. There's a saying that you should 'sleep when you're tired, eat when you're hungry', and that's all you've got to do. You don't go to sleep in the middle of the afternoon because you're bored, and you don't go to sleep mid-morning because you've had a row with someone, so why would you eat in these situations?

When you do a day's gardening, or something similarly strenuous, and really put your back into it, you might finish the day with a long hot bath and an early night. The sleep following muscular exhaustion – when you're really tired – is a deep, wonderful, relaxing sleep. That's exactly the same as sitting down and eating a meal when you *actually need it,* rather than when the clock says it's a particular time. If you sit down and eat a succulent steak or lobster when you're really hungry, it'll be amazing. When you eat it for no other reason than because it's 7 p.m. and therefore 'dinner time', it'll have a completely different appeal[9] – try it sometime.

All of this is, of course, why there are so many overweight children today. Eating whether they're hungry or not. There should be no place in society for behaviour like this. In fact, there was some public debate about whether parents who feed their children a diet consisting mainly of junk food, ready meals and processed foods, resulting in the youngsters becoming obese, should be made to take nutrition education classes.

If you're not hungry, why are you eating? Are you so sad that all you can do in your life is stuff food in your mouth? Can't you go for a walk? Paint a picture? Read a book? Watch a film? Look at the sunset?

People are eating for all the wrong reasons, and many are eating themselves to death.

*'I realized I'd never been truly hungry… I've cut down on portion sizes and now I feel full **before** I finish. The most important lesson I've learned is that food and drink don't have to control your life. You should control them. I can't thank Martin and Marion enough for changing my life so dramatically.'*
GMB CLIENT **C.W.**

Are You Ready for the Next Step?

So, you've been overeating for years – maybe all your adult life. Now things are going to change. You know that looking and feeling good comes at a price, and that price is a bit of effort – the slim person knows that. Eating healthily, eating what your body needs, may require a bit of effort, but it isn't a punishment!

Later in the book, you'll read some GMB clients' personal weight-loss stories, and probably recognize many of the feelings they admit to having had when they were overweight. They know only too well how the weight loss–gain cycle leads to a feeling of hopelessness. What they'll tell you very clearly though is that the GMB therapy has turned their lives around, and completely altered their relationship with food.

Overweight people wear their problems for all to see in the shape of their bodies. For those with other issues – drug addiction, alcoholism or severe depression, for example – the problem isn't usually visible when they walk down the street.

When you work through the four GMB sessions in Part 2 of the book, you'll see the ways in which you make the wrong food choices; the times when you eat for the wrong reason; and the different triggers you have that have led you down the road to obesity. Better still, the sessions will show you there's a fork in that road, and that you're standing there right now, about to make the choice that will lead to a totally different, manageable – and enjoyable – relationship with food.

IN THIS BOOK YOU'LL LEARN:

- About the psychology of overeating.
- To recognize your own personal triggers.
- To question *why* you eat.
- How to identify your motivation for losing excess weight.
- How to understand hunger.
- The differences between need, desire and craving.
- Why you can show restraint in other areas of your life but not with food.
- How thirst can be mistaken for hunger.
- How to remain positive over a long-term weight loss.

Chapter 3
Anyone for Gastric Band Surgery?

Have you ever thought about having gastric band surgery? If so, you not alone. Every year, thousands of people not only think about it, but actually do it. Statistics vary, but there's no doubt that the number of obese individuals has risen hugely in the past 20 years, and bariatric surgery is a solution to the problem that is being used more and more. However, even people who've had a gastric band fitted acknowledge that it's far from the miracle 'cure' they expect it to be.

Surgical gastric bands were first developed by a Ukrainian, Dr Lubomyr Kuzmak, in the early 1980s. By 1986 Kuzmak had implanted an adjustable silicone gastric band to address severe obesity. Obesity surgeon Professor Franco Favretti's team then adopted Kuzmak's system, and between 1991 and 1994 more than 2,000 gastric bands were implanted, although the system was not suitable for laparoscopic ('keyhole surgery') procedures. Trials and tests for an adjustable laparoscopic band were completed by 1993, and the first two were implanted in Belgium and Italy that year. US trials started in 1995, but the system didn't receive US approval until 2001.

Gastric bands are usually only offered to patients with a BMI of over 40, or a BMI of 35–40 if they have other health problems such as heart disease, high blood pressure or diabetes.[1] A typical gastric band operation involves placing an adjustable silicone band around the upper part of the stomach to create a pouch. The band's tightness is adjusted by injections of a saline solution into a port located just below the patient's skin.

As the subject eats, the pouch fills much more quickly than their stomach would, because it's a fraction of the size – about the size of a golf ball rather than the 1-litre (1.75-pint) capacity of an un-stretched stomach. As a result, the subject can generally eat far smaller quantities than they could without the band. This is designed to reduce the number of calories consumed and lead to weight loss.

From the pouch, the food passes slowly into the lower part of the stomach, through a narrow adjustable opening created by the band, and then usually through the rest of the digestive system.

The operation involves making between one and five incisions in the patient's upper abdomen; the band is fitted via keyhole surgery lasting between 30 minutes and one hour. Gas is pumped into the abdominal cavity to make space for the surgeon's equipment during the procedure. The band is held in place within the patient's body with stitches. The initial incisions from surgery are closed with two or three stitches.

A fine tube runs from the band to an access point or 'port' secured under the skin around the chest/ribs, or sometimes the abdomen area. A few weeks after surgery, the band is adjusted by injecting precise quantities of saline through the skin into the port, and via the tube, to 'inflate' the band. There are often two or three adjustments – each requiring repeat hospital or clinic visits – in the first few months after the operation.

This, however, is a very basic description of the process. What happens before and after the operation is currently not fully understood by the general public. You are obese, you get a gastric band fitted, you can't eat very much, you lose weight, right? And you lose it faster/better/more easily than any other reversible method, don't you?

Gastric Band Surgery: The Full Story

The reality is rather different, and it all starts several weeks before the operation itself. Patients are instructed to start following a strict diet to ensure that the liver – which sits above and partly in front of the stomach – is not too fatty. Having an enlarged liver is a problem commonly associated with overeating.

In gastric band surgery, the liver has to be moved to one side for the operation to take place, and if it's enlarged, it can literally get in the way, as well as increasing the risk of serious damage to it during the procedure. In fact, it has been known for part of the liver to break off during surgery, leading to massive internal haemorrhaging.

Depending on the surgeon, the patient's pre-op diet is a restricted one, low in sugar, fat and carbohydrates. With each 28g (1oz) of glycogen (a form of sugar stored in the liver, and in muscles for energy) the body also stores 85–133g (3–4oz) of water, so for patients on this strict diet, low in starch and sugar, the body loses glycogen and water, thus shrinking the liver.

Having followed a strict eating regime before they even reach the operating theatre, gastric band surgery patients often lose up to a stone (6.3kg) or more by reducing the amount of food they eat.

Once the band's in place, the soups and blended foods the patient is advised to eat after surgery give the swollen stomach a bit of a rest. How long this diet lasts varies, but it can be for about six weeks, so the weight continues to drop because the patient has gone from eating massive quantities (despite what people often say, it is *extremely* rare to become overweight without eating far more than your body needs) to following a restrictive diet for three weeks, then living on soup for another six weeks.

Work it out. Before the band comes into play, the patient will have lost anything up to 1st 6lbs (9kg). No surgery, just sensible eating!

At six weeks post-op, the patient has their first 'fill' of the band. Saline solution is injected via the port, inflating the band to reduce the outlet and restrict the flow of food. It may take quite a lot of adjustment – everyone's different – so the medical team gets the patient to try to eat and drink while they're doing it to check if it's right. If it's too restrictive, they may not even be able to drink water in case they vomit it all up. The surgical team must get it exactly right so the patient can eat little bits and feel the restriction, but not to the point where they can't get anything down.

When a 'bandster' or 'bandit' (as gastric band patients dub themselves) has the right amount of fluid in their band so their weight is coming down steadily, they refer to this as finding their 'sweet spot'.

After the first fill the patient is slowly reintroduced to solid foods, though their meal size is still around six tablespoons (90ml) of food. Return visits to the clinic or hospital are required as often as necessary to have the fill adjusted to ensure continued weight loss. Obviously the weight loss is quite fast to begin with, but once it's settled down, the figure overall, according to the World Health Organization (WHO), averages out at between 1–2lb (0.45–0.90kg) per week, which is no different from any sensible weight-loss programme.

This simply replicates what GMB would expect to achieve. You shouldn't lose any more than that over an extended period of time anyway – not least because rapid weight loss can lead to the development of gallstones.

So, the surgical gastric band only offers the same long-term weight loss as any surgery-free healthy eating plan. And it's not foolproof. The success rate is only 70 per cent; in all likelihood, the main reason for it not being 100 per cent is because patients can cheat on the band by how they eat. Obviously solid foods will stay in the pouch for a long time, making it harder to overeat because of discomfort once the pouch is full, but softer things –ice cream, chocolate, etc. – will pass through quite quickly. These are referred to as 'slider foods', for obvious reasons.

**Bandsters' experiences, good and bad,
are easily found on forums if you care
to look online for yourself!**

So, if you were a comfort eater before the surgery, and prefer foods that don't take a lot of chewing before they disintegrate, you could still go through life drip-feeding yourself on mashed-up junk food – softened chocolate, ice cream etc. – and the band won't actively restrict it at all. The same applies to alcohol, which as you'll learn when we discuss portion control and calories, is like drinking calories that are no use to your body whatsoever – they are just 'empty' calories. If you like to drink water during a meal, that's not advised after gastric band surgery because it frees up the food matter to pass out of the pouch more easily. So you don't feel full for as long as you would do without the water.

What Are the Risks?

So, do you want to know what you'd be putting your body through, and the potential risks and downsides of gastric band surgery? What follows is a brief overview, taken from the British Obesity Surgery Patient Association (BOSPA) website,[2] and other sources.

There are risks involved in any surgery when the patient is under general anaesthesia. These range from infection and unexpected reaction to the anaesthetic, to developing a blood clot, an allergic reaction to substances leading to cardiovascular problems, jaundice, and slow recovery due to poor heart, liver or kidney function. And, of course, being obese makes undergoing any surgery intrinsically more risky.

Approximately 1 in 100 patients develop serious complications following gastric band surgery.[3] A report produced by researchers at Florida's Mount Sinai Medical Center's Department of Surgery says that severely obese patients are at increased risk of pulmonary embolism, wound infection and other complications.[4]

Obesity makes it hard for surgeons and medical teams to establish whether the patient has underlying health problems; aches and pains might be due to their weight, or indicative of a more serious problem. For example, chest tightness may be caused by an underlying cardiac problem, or simply due to their obesity.

> *'Undergoing surgery to assist with weight loss*
> *is a serious procedure, not a quick fix.'*
> PROFESSOR PETER LITTLEJOHNS, NATIONAL INSTITUTE FOR HEALTH AND
> CLINICAL EXCELLENCE **(NICE)** WEIGHT-LOSS SURGERY APPRAISAL LEADER.

The patient has to fast for about six hours before having a general anaesthetic, and must sign a consent form confirming they understand the risks, as well as the benefits, of the procedure. They may have to wear compression stockings to help prevent blood clots in the veins in their legs, and they may also need an injection of anti-clotting medicine.

Once the operation is complete, the patient rests until the effects of the anaesthesia have passed, and then they may need some or all of the following: pain relief, a catheter in their bladder (if you've had one, you'll know how uncomfortable this is), tubes to drain their wound(s), fluids via a drip, a post-operative x-ray to check the position of the band, and compression pads on their legs.

Patients return home after about a day and have to drink clear fluids for the first 24 hours. They then start on other liquids, leading on to pureed foods (like baby food) for a few weeks.

There's a follow-up appointment to check that the wounds are healing, followed by several repeat visits for band adjustments. The amount of time the stitches remain in place depends on whether they're soluble or not — they'll disappear on their own in 7–10 days if they are. If they aren't, it means another hospital/clinic visit for them to be removed. Patients shouldn't drive for about a fortnight after the operation, and a full recovery from its effects can take three weeks.

After an initial drastic weight loss in the first nine weeks or so, the average loss for someone who's had gastric band surgery is 5–10lb (2.26–4.5kg) per month.

Side Effects and Complications

Here are some of the possible things that can go wrong, during and after surgery:

- Post-anaesthesia sickness; bruising; pain; swelling of the skin around the wound sites; feeling or actually being sick after eating; and requiring multivitamin supplements because of the restricted diet. If the patient is unlucky enough to get an infection that doesn't respond to antibiotics, the band may have to be removed.

- There could be damage to other organs in the abdomen caused during the operation, or slippage – months or even years after the operation, there's always the risk that the stomach will move up through the band and the upper pouch will become enlarged. (The band can be re-fixed in the correct position.)

- Leakage – this may be due to damage of the reservoir or tubing if fills are not carried out with extreme care, or if two of the band components come apart. Again, this would necessitate replacement of the damaged component.

- Erosion – very slowly, and particularly if the adjustment balloon is tightly inflated, the band can work its way into or through the wall of the stomach and cease to be effective. In this case the band would be removed and replaced, if possible. The band itself is made of silicone, and there are no known side effects to this material inside the body. However, it's possible that, at some time in the future, the band may need to be replaced simply because it's worn out. Or that newer, better bands have been developed to replace current ones.

- Gallstones – these sometimes develop if one loses weight quickly, and can require surgery to remove them. In fact, some surgeons advise removing the entire gallbladder at the same time as having gastric band surgery.

- Occasionally a surgeon converts from a keyhole procedure to open surgery, which requires a bigger cut on the abdomen.

- Acid reflux – many 'bandsters' seem to regard this side effect as the norm, but in bad cases, people can experience burning sensations in their throat as a result of the simple act of lying down in bed at night.

- And finally, as many as 60 per cent of gastric band patients may need a 'repair' or a replacement band.[5] Others, having regained the weight lost, may be recommended to have the far more serious, and usually irreversible, gastric bypass surgery.

There are three other key points:

- Provision of the Adjustable Gastric Band is generally limited to people between the ages of 18 and 55 with a BMI over 40 (over 35 if there are additional health issues). In the USA it's a BMI of 30–40 with at least one additional health issue.

- As we explained earlier, because people can 'cheat' the band, and, unless they've gone through psychological steps to change their relationship with food, it's not always the miracle cure they hoped for.

- In practice, many gastric band providers look at figures of between 50 and 60 per cent of excess weight lost over two years, but did you realize that with the Adjustable Gastric Band, success is not defined as reaching your 'desirable', 'goal', or 'proper' weight, but as losing more than 25 per cent of your excess weight.[6]

So you could be 5ft 6in (1.68m) tall, weigh 224lb (101.6kg) with a BMI of 36.2, aiming at around 152lb (68.9kg) to achieve a healthy BMI of 24.5. You could have a band fitted, lose 18lb (8kg) and be considered a success story – whereas in fact you'd be someone 5ft 6in tall, still weighing 206lb (93.4kg), still with a raised BMI (about 33 – obese) and still wishing you were a good 45lb (20kg) or more lighter.

Okay, so you've got the band fitted – what now? According to the British Obesity Surgery Patient Association (BOSPA), there are six golden eating-plan rules to follow if you're dedicated to obtaining the greatest benefit from your gastric band:[7]

- Eat three meals per day.

- Eat healthy, solid food.

- Eat slowly and stop as soon as you feel full.

- Don't eat between meals.

- Don't drink at mealtimes.

- All drinks should contain zero calories.

They suggest eating a healthy balanced diet, including foods from each of the five main food groups. Several foods aren't tolerated well, or can cause blockages and/or vomiting. These include oranges, meat (this needs to be chopped to the size of an end-of-pencil rubber before considerable chewing), broccoli, dried fruit, coconut, crisps, nuts, popcorn, soft white bread, pineapple, asparagus, and more.

So, you could say that the eating plan with a surgical gastric band is: eat nutritious food slowly, and don't graze or snack between meals. Think about it — if you did that anyway, you wouldn't need the band in the first place!

A Few More Facts

Here are some other things to consider about gastric band surgery:

- If you have to pay for your own operation, the cost can be high — think upwards of £3,500, plus accommodation.

- If the patient is advised to have their gallbladder removed because of the increased risk of developing gallstones, they might suffer from bloating, indigestion, constipation or diarrhoea. They could also develop stones in the liver, which cause congestion.

- It's not unknown for the liver, or another organ, to be accidently perforated during surgery because of how tightly packed together all the organs are in the abdomen.

- An overfilled band can lead to choking.

- Bands can erode into the stomach wall. If this happens they need to be removed and gastric bypass considered as an alternative solution. This involves stapling across the top of the stomach, removing a portion of the small intestine and reattaching it. However, the first part of the small intestine is where the body absorbs nutrients, so patients have to take supplements afterwards.

- With less intestinal tract for food to travel down, people with a gastric bypass can experience uncontrollable diarrhoea (the so-called Dumping Syndrome) after consuming rich foods.

- The band may need several tightening sessions. The adjustment of the band can be complex, involving maybe only an extra 1ml (0.035 fl oz) of saline each time. Once at the optimum level (the sweet spot), it's not adjusted again until the target is reached, after which the band can be loosened slightly to aim for weight maintenance rather than loss.

- If a patient vomits repeatedly, their retching can loosen the band from its stitches, leading to further surgery for repositioning.

- Going from overeating to only eating about 6 tablespoons (90ml) of food per plate is a huge adjustment; the bandster needs to chew each mouthful of food at least 10 times.

- The feeling of fullness is higher up in the chest with a gastric band, leading to chest pain that is indigestion, but which often gets confused with heart problems.

- If the sphincter muscle at the top of the stomach doesn't work properly, any acid build-up in the stomach can come back up into the oesophagus, causing a burning sensation. This is called acid reflux, and happens because of the small quantities of food in the lower part of the stomach. The rest is in the pouch, drip-feeding through.

- With an over-tightened band, someone may not even be able to swallow a mouthful of water without regurgitating it.

- As yet, research into the long-term implications of gastric band surgery is limited.

In conclusion, then, if you've got your head sorted out, you shouldn't actually need to have this foreign body inside you for the rest of your life! You are relying on the band to do the whole job, rather than relying on your mind. It's much better to get your mindset right.

Having the operation doesn't help you build a better relationship with food, either; it's just like a diet in which you end up even more obsessed with food. You'll be forever thinking, *Is that mouthful too big? Did I chew that mouthful 10 times before I swallowed it? Oh no, I haven't left a long enough gap between eating and drinking!*

Imagine how difficult and uncomfortable it would be going to a restaurant with friends. To try to sit down and eat a meal in front of them, with all these things you'd have to consider. You'd always feel on edge.

That said, there's no doubt that the gastric band procedure has been life changing for many people. It's *relatively* safe and is now being carried out in most countries in the world. For some, maybe many, it has been a lifesaver.

As a postscript, it's worth noting that there are no intrinsic dangers or side effects from any elements of the Gastric Mind Band treatment. And, of course, there is no invasive surgery.

LINDA'S STORY

If ever there was a cautionary tale about surgical gastric bands, it's that of GMB client Linda, who went through two life-threatening band failures and excruciating abdominal pain over a period of almost two years because she remained convinced that the band – by then going severely wrong – was the answer to her weight problem.

The 31-year-old, 5ft 4in (1.63m) mother-of-three wasn't sure what she weighed – somewhere around 21 stone (133kg). But, as she was wearing size 26 and 28 clothes, she knew one thing: her target was a size 10/12, and she believed the only way she'd achieve it was through surgery.

'I was huge,' Linda recalls. 'I'd just given birth to my son and I knew I couldn't go through another year of getting bigger. I had to do something drastic. But, with what I know now, I wouldn't recommend the band to anyone. At times I had pain like I'd never had in my life.'

Linda decided on a gastric band after thorough research. 'In the end I felt there were too many things that could go wrong with a gastric bypass,' she says. 'At the time I thought the band was the best thing since sliced bread. I was told it was virtually pain-free; that I'd ache a bit after surgery, but could expect to be up on my feet within a couple of days. That sounded perfect. I had a baby and two other children, and I was constantly doing school runs.'

The cost of the surgery started out at just under £8,700, but it rose to £10,500 with repeat visits for fills. But

Linda was more than happy once the weight started dropping off. 'Once I'd booked in I had to slash my food intake for two weeks to shrink my liver, so I was on three low-calorie diet drinks a day and shifted a stone (6.3kg),' she says. 'But I felt really ill because I was used to such a high intake of calories. By the time I went in for the operation I'd lost about 2.5 stone (16kg) on my own.'

Linda was in considerable pain when she came round from the surgery, but, despite being booked in for three nights in hospital, she was sent home the following day, told that it was to get her moving to avoid developing blood clots. 'I had the band fitted just three months after having my baby, and now I think it was too soon,' she says. 'I don't think my stomach was really ready. I should have waited a year. At the time I was so desperate that it wouldn't have mattered what any of the doctors said… except they didn't, because my mum made a point of asking them.'

Linda's recovery didn't go well from the outset. 'I felt absolutely awful. I couldn't pick anything up – it was excruciating. I started getting on my feet in the second week, but I wasn't pain free,' she says. Then followed the trial and error of discovering what she could and couldn't eat.

'You're tender, and while you're trying things out you try not to be sick because you could hurt yourself. For me, everything would bounce back up again. I had to eat very slowly: very small pieces, very small quantities. A coaster-sized plate as a meal; mashed carrots and swede for example. Toddler food really. It was very hard work. I wasn't feeling well, but I didn't care because I was losing weight. I just wanted to be able to go into a clothes shop and pick something off the shelf – that was my dream, what I was focused on.

'I was being really good because I'd paid all that money. Through the support group I heard about people who ate chips and melted-down Mars bars, and I thought, why? Why have you got to the point of undergoing surgery yet you still want to eat this stuff and then sit there saying you haven't lost a lot of weight.'

From Bad to Worse

One weekend it became obvious that things weren't as they should be. 'I felt really ill; I'd drink and feel sick, and I just couldn't eat,' Linda remembers. 'I'd have a sip of water and it would come back up. Then, even putting water on my tongue would make me gag. I couldn't hold myself up, and my husband had to carry me to the toilet. I could barely speak.'

Luckily for Linda, someone from the support group suggested a barium test. 'I got an emergency appointment, and was told I was very lucky – my organs were shutting down because the band had somehow tightened. I was told the chances were high that I could've gone into a coma, possibly died. As soon as they loosened the band off, it was fine. At the time I was told this was the first case they'd ever had, but despite trying to consult my specialist about why this had happened, no further action was taken.'

So Linda had the band adjusted, and, despite her misgivings about what might happen if it tightened again, she got on with her life and her continued weight loss.

But, several months later, the same thing happened again. 'They didn't have a clue why – nothing had triggered it, but there seemed to be no research. At that point the hospital hadn't had a band that had gone wrong. Obviously these occasions made me very ill; I couldn't do anything, and so my husband had to look after me and take the children to and from school. This meant he couldn't work, so we were losing even more money.'

Linda suffered from bad heartburn and was sometimes sick in her sleep. 'That is absolutely terrifying,' she says. 'Your natural instinct is to swallow, but you can't for fear of choking!' She carried on with the discomfort, but two years later she still felt really ill. 'I'd got to the stage where every time I drank or ate I got excruciating pains in my upper back – if I ate too much of something it felt like I was swallowing it "down my back" – but I didn't know how or why.

'I got a cough, my chest hurt, everything hurt. I had tests, but I was convinced it wasn't the band… it was a completely different feeling. Antibiotics didn't touch it. It got really bad, and in the end I paid to go back to the consultant, which I begrudged. He said it couldn't be the band.'

The Bombshell News

Linda eventually had an endoscopy and it was revealed that her band had tightened and gone through her stomach wall and into her top bowel. *How could this possibly happen?* she thought. 'I'd only just finished paying. It was really selfish of me; I wasn't even thinking about what was going on inside me. I was about 10 stone (63.6kg) then, and wearing size 10 jeans. I was devastated.'

She was told that the band had to come out as soon as possible, and that it would be possible to insert a 'slip' – like a small-scale bypass. But, ultimately, the risks of doing this were too great. 'When I came round, I experienced pain like I've never felt in my entire life,' Linda says. 'I was all wired up, tubes in my mouth and nose and everything. I lay there and honestly thought I'd died. Then my chest drains were left in for too long and they fused in to my ribs; I had to spend five days in hospital.

'At home recovering, I got a serious infection. I'd been feverish and hallucinating and one day I got upstairs in agony, bent over to do something, heard a "pop" and a load of yellow pus and blood poured out of wounds on my chest.'

Linda went down the road of investigating compensation, or at least seeing if she could persuade anyone to highlight her problems. 'I did all the complaining I could, but I hit a brick wall. A solicitor advised me that going to court would cost a great deal of money, and that it would have been the first case of its kind she had dealt with.'

She traced other cases in the USA, where most patients have gone on to have another band fitted or a gastric bypass. 'I was told there was too much damage to have another band fitted,' Linda says with a rueful smile.

Today, she is still restricted as to what she can eat: 'I find it hard at times to drink and eat together: that brings on the feeling of suffocation.' She also has occasional breathlessness, back pain and pain in the area where the port was. 'After the surgery, for the first time I had the feeling that food didn't rule me, but I paid a big price for it – three near-death experiences. It's a high price to pay, both financially and with your health. I'm lucky I'm here to tell my story. I wouldn't recommend the band to anyone.'

Before Linda had GMB therapy, she'd given up. 'I felt I'd been failed by the system, and I was really low. I'd regained much of the weight I'd lost, and I just wanted someone to wave a magic wand. Once I met Marion and Martin, though, I was upbeat from the start. Although I gave in to a few temptations that Christmas, with what I learned with GMB I got back on track quickly and couldn't wait to get to the gym. Something had changed!

'I'm hopeful this is going to "cure" me of my bad relationship with food… I want to not have the nagging voice in the back of my mind day in, day out, arguing with myself as to whether I should eat all that pizza or just half of it, and so on. To have a better understanding. With GMB I know I'll be feeling on top of the world again.

'I've already changed. My life now includes exercise every day, and it's not a chore. It makes me feel good. The best thing is not being on a diet. This is a lifestyle. There are no forbidden foods. Have anything but in moderation; don't beat yourself up about it, just pick yourself up and carry on. If you've decided something on your own – say to have a salad instead of a sandwich – you feel so good. I can't believe it's actually me saying this, but it's really how I feel. I'm in control – at last!'

WHAT YOU'VE LEARNED IN THIS CHAPTER

- A gastric band is a successful way for some people to lose excess weight.
- It's relatively easy to 'cheat' the gastric band.
- The weight loss achieved with a surgical gastric band may not be any greater than that achieved by following a healthy eating plan.
- Even if you do your research, there are no guarantees that the band will work for you.
- Gastric bands can and do go wrong.
- GMB therapy can offer new hope.

Chapter 4
Developing the Gastric Mind Band

As we explained earlier in the book, the idea for the Gastric Mind Band came up purely by chance when a client we'd successfully helped give up smoking using hypnotherapy had begun to gain weight. She had a friend who'd just had a gastric band fitted at a cost of £11,000, and, since she didn't want to spend thousands herself (and it was an operation she didn't want), she asked if we could just hypnotize her again, this time into believing she'd had the operation!

At the time, it just seemed like a joke, and we thought no more about it. However, that evening we had to fly back to the UK, and at the airport, over a glass of wine, we started talking about it. Marion's reaction to the idea was: why not? By the time we arrived in the UK, we'd exhausted the laptop battery and filled several A4 sheets of paper with an outline proposal for a treatment package that would conclude with the fitting of an *imaginary* gastric band. Effectively, by then we felt there was a good chance we could do exactly what our client had suggested. As time went on, we sculpted, added to and refined our thoughts and ideas, and developed the GMB therapy – the subject of ongoing research and development even today.

Our Guinea Pig

Martin was our lead guinea pig – he was the obvious candidate because he was overweight himself. As things progressed, though, we had an ever-growing list of clients and friends all prepared – some very keen, in fact – to help with the trials.

At first we tried just hypnotherapy, but we found it too light, and of limited success. We then tried just using CBT, but on its own that didn't cut it. Next we tried hypnotherapy together with NLP, but that didn't work in the permanent way we were looking for either. Gradually, over the course of the following 18 months, all three approaches were used to underpin one another. Putting the three therapies together in this way ticked all the boxes and did the job. We'd come up with the Gastric Mind Band treatment using our own mix of therapies that we called Life Architecture. Being the architect of your own life is, after all, your birthright.

In order to get the most from the hypnotherapy sessions, we knew we had to engage clients' senses, so we developed techniques and used devices that would enable us to introduce the sounds and smells of the garden and beach during the relaxation into a hypnotic state. We added ways to include the taste of sea salt on clients' lips, and the smell of ozone; we then helped them to experience the sights, sounds and smells of the hospital, and, ultimately, the gastric band 'operating theatre'.

When experienced in real life, those sensations are really memorable; during therapy, the client gets the most from it if the virtual reality is as accurate as possible.

This book can never replace one-on-one hypnotherapy, or treatment as experienced in the clinic. However, if you are sufficiently motivated, you will be as focused, and as receptive to the suggestions we'll be making to you, as if you were sitting in front of us.

There was really only one way to be sure whether the Gastric Mind Band worked – Martin tried it himself. At the start of the trials for our new therapy, Martin weighed in at 18st 12lb (120kg). Seven months later, he was 13st 1lb (83kg), with an 86-cm (34-in) waist. A loss of 81lb (37kg). As we have done with all our 'case studies', we asked Martin to tell us his weight history.

MARTIN SHIRRAN'S STORY

'When I was about 11 years old, I had to see the school doctor every couple of months,' Martin says. 'I remember I was 7 stone 7lb (47.7kg) – it never changed. I was thin and I stayed that way for a long time.

'By the time I was 16, though, I was what I suppose you'd call overweight, and while I dieted on and off over the years, nothing really changed. I would lose a couple of stone and then put on three. My brother and sister were never thin, but they didn't seem to be uncomfortable with their weight; my dad was a normal weight, and so was my mum until later in her life.

'At my heaviest I must have been getting close to 19 stone (121kg). My weight had been a problem for nearly as long as I could remember. I was never really depressed about it, although I went through phases of trying to do something about it. However, I think that while being overweight is certainly an issue for men, it has a different priority level to how women feel about it.

'Everyone who goes through the GMB treatment seems to benefit in different ways from the various sections and approaches. For me, the CBT – understanding the psychological reasons why I ate, and how I thought about food – is the part that has stayed with me the longest. Of course, as time has gone on, I've developed new approaches – not just for myself, but for the many clients I now see each week.

'I have lived with the trials and discussions, sometimes 24/7. What worked the best? The whole thing. But in particular I'm now more in tune with my body than perhaps I have ever been in my adult life. I can now recognize hunger, *real* hunger. I live by the rule 'sleep when you are tired, eat only when you are hungry'. It works for me.

'I know that clients' views differ on the overall importance of the 'operation' element of the therapy, but it definitely played a part for me. It does underpin everything we do.'

Martin now eats and drinks differently, and for different reasons. 'I look at everything and everybody differently now,' he says. 'I've tried to work out why, when a certain couple visited us in the UK, we, or more truthfully I, would end up drinking more alcohol than I should have. I was questioning why it always happened with the same couple. Then it came to me: I think they bored me – their conversation wasn't stimulating, and so I was therefore self-prescribing, self-medicating, with what I believed was an anti-depressant, namely alcohol.

'The tools that have helped me, and those that I still use today, include identifying the Diet Terrorists: those people who manage, often without any effort, to create total chaos in the lives of people trying to practise healthy weight control. Here are some examples of what I mean.'

Watching Out for the Diet Terrorists

'Sometimes, on our way home from the clinic, Marion and I visit a local Chinese restaurant, usually planning to have just one course between us. All is fine; unless, that is, the owner's daughter serves us. Before the menu arrives, she sends over a complimentary, extra-large portion of prawn crackers. We never order them, and we're never sure whether we actually want them, but there they are, right under our noses. If I have just one, I know I'm at risk of blowing my eating plan for the night. It's hard to have just one prawn cracker, wouldn't you agree?

'Of course, this lady is highly trained in the art of chaos; it's as if she sees us getting out of the car and plans the whole thing: no one else gets jumbo-sized portions of crackers for free, just us. Whether I manage to get past the prawn crackers or not matters very little – this girl's good, very good! When the bill comes at the end of the meal it's always presented at the table along with two complimentary drinks from the bar, and they're always the same thing: Baileys. I always think that she must say "gotcha" as we walk out the door. The prawn crackers before we even get the menu, those two Baileys – that's 900 calories.

'Once, we joined some friends for an Indian meal. I was determined to drink only water, and to only order a chicken tikka starter served as a main course – no rice or

Indian bread. We sat down, and before I'd even pulled my chair in, the waiter brought over a tray piled high with about 24 poppadums and put them in the middle of the table. "Who ordered those?" I asked. "They're free," was the reply. Great! The waiter returned two minutes later with a tray of chutneys as well. There were six of us and he could have put the tray anywhere on the table, but he chose, of course, to put it right in front of me. Diet Terrorist, or what!?

'Another time, when visiting my 90-year-old mum, I'd sat down for a cup of tea when she said, "I bought some of your favourite biscuits; go and put a few on a plate." I haven't eaten biscuits for 10 years, but what could I say? When I opened her kitchen cupboard it was full of boxes of biscuits. Why had she bought enough to feed an army? They were on a two-for-one offer at the supermarket, she told me, so she'd bought a dozen extra packets for me to take back to Spain. "I remember that years ago you used to love them, so I thought I'd treat you," she said. Another terrorist: my mum!

'Then, at a friend's mother's for Sunday lunch, I spent most of the time in the kitchen talking to her while she cooked. It proved to be an education. We were having roast beef with all the trimmings. As we chatted, she'd opened the oven, but only to baste the beef and the roast potatoes. It was at that point that I realized that accepting this invitation may not have been such a good idea.

'The meat was being cooked in an oven tin, which was standing on a baking rack to allow the fat to drain off. My friend's mum ladled all the fat that had just been drained from the beef back over it again. Then she poured the remainder of the fat over the potatoes. Over the next hour or so, I watched in amazement as she re-opened the oven three more times and re-poured the fat over the meat and potatoes. The reason people like roast potatoes so much is because of all the fat used to crisp up the outsides!

'Then, before the meal, she took the tin from the oven, the fat still in the bottom, and put it on the stove. She then sprinkled some granules in it and made a fat-based gravy to pour over everyone's healthy, fresh, organically grown vegetables.'

Staying on Track
'The Pause Button technique, which you can use to 'freeze' time, gives you precious moments to ensure you make the right decision, having weighed up the consequences. I use it on a daily basis, along with the fork in the road described later. Both have been invaluable to me, and I use them in many other situations, not just those relating to food. So can you. (The method is explained later, in Chapter 11.)

'Before, my eating patterns hadn't been good – too many of the wrong foods, eating late at night and usually skipping breakfast. I now eat a light, healthy breakfast every day, often just fresh fruits, and I try to have my last meal of the day as early as possible.

'I started to lose weight straight away – quite quickly to begin with, and then, as I expected, it gradually slowed down. I had a few plateaux along the way; I know how hard they can be, but I carried on, sometimes changing my diet, sometimes the time of day that I ate my main meal, and sometimes generally increasing my exercise level.

'I remember a period of three weeks when I thought it had all gone wrong, and I was close to throwing my toys out of the pram! I'd been regularly losing between 1 and 1.5lb (0.45–0.68kg) a week. Then, one Monday at my regular weekly weigh-in, I'd lost nothing. My food intake had been on track and consistent, as had my exercise level. I insisted that Marion change the batteries in the scales. She did so – reluctantly! Same recording, same result. Somehow though, she convinced me to carry on.

'She reminded me of all the hard work I'd put in – the fantastic results we'd achieved week on week – and how good I felt about myself. So I carried on, and the next week when I was weighed I'd put on 1lb (0.45kg). I doubt whether anyone other than someone familiar with long-term weight loss will ever know just how depressed I felt at that stage. I gave it one last week, and of course I then found I was back on track!'

As for 'overriding' the Gastric Mind Band, Martin says he was able to adopt the 'some meals matter, some don't' way of thinking (see page 179) over Christmas – pre-planning it and relaxing the tension over the holiday period. So, does he believe the Gastric Mind Band part of the treatment? 'Absolutely. One hundred and ten per cent.'

Two notable episodes in Martin's journey happened on the same day. 'At the airport, we were sharing a table with a couple and their two children, and one of them spilled a chocolate milkshake over me,' he recalls. 'Marion said, "Why not just go over and buy a new pair of jeans?" I ran over to a shop, picked up a pair of 83-cm (33-in) waist jeans and put them on. I couldn't remember the last time I'd been able to choose a pair of jeans off the rail. Anyone who is overweight knows the significance of such an event.

'An hour or so later, on the flight, we bought a couple of drinks and the stewardess leaned over and undid my tray catch and put mine on it. It was amazing – not only to have the tray down with drinks on it, but also to have a space between my stomach and the tray! It was only a small thing, but you did ask.'

WHAT YOU'VE LEARNED IN THIS CHAPTER

- It's the mix of therapies in GMB – the Life Architecture – that makes the difference.
- If you're motivated, anything is achievable.
- Although the results will never be identical, you can get a very similar experience to our Gastric Mind Band clinical therapy by reading this book, and reinforcing the key elements through self-hypnosis.
- A plateau is a plateau, nothing more. Work through it.

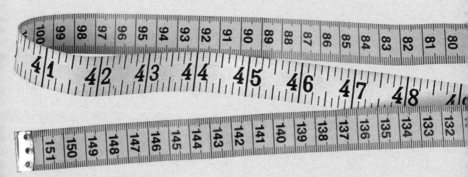

PART 2
YOUR STORY

Chapter 5
The Sessions: A Life-Changing Sequence

The Gastric Mind Band therapy is actually a process of learning about yourself and your flawed eating patterns, and then unlocking the underlying reasons why and how these have developed. It involves learning new eating habits, understanding how to make better food choices, and living the rest of your life with a healthier relationship with food.

At the clinics, the treatment is carried out over four sessions. These are made up of 12 hours of therapy – usually over four consecutive days – concluding with the unique Gastric Mind Band element. Our clients find that the various parts of the four sessions affect them in different ways. As you read this book, you'll pick up those specific anecdotes, rules, thoughts or observations that 'get to you' more successfully than others.

There are so many of these that sometimes you'll think they're being repeated. They are; sometimes with slight adjustments. It's no bad thing to be reminded in as many ways as possible of just how you've been tricking yourself – cheating yourself, allowing your mind to give you the go-ahead for all sorts of behaviours that have ended up with you overweight, unhappy and looking for help to get out of the mess you're in.

The Gastric Mind Band Experience

Everyone reads a book in the way they choose to, but with this one, if you can keep to reading it in the order in which it's been written – retracing your steps as and when necessary – you'll make the best progress. The sessions, in particular, run in a sequence – identifying your problems with food, identifying when, how and how much you should be eating, spotting the errors you've been making, and ultimately, capping the process off with the 'fitting' of the Gastric Mind Band. The progression is obvious, and you'll make the most of your experience if you can work through the sessions logically.

Session 1

In the clinic, this lasts for up to four hours. It starts with the client being weighed, and their body composition being analyzed for fat mass, body fat percentage, visceral fat, muscle mass and BMI. After the treatment is explained, this session is all about building up a picture of the client – by harvesting personal information, poking with awkward questions, creating a personalized history – and keeping a record of their full story. We ask them, and now you in the next chapter, 'Why do you eat?', 'Why are you overweight?' and 'Isn't it tiring carrying all those extra calories and pounds of fat around?' We ensure that they start to question everything they eat, everything they put in their mouths.

Hypnosis and Visualization

The session ends with a 20-minute hypnosis session in which the client is asked to visualize a fork in the road; another year overweight, not liking themselves and feeling sad. Probably getting fatter. Or the other route: visualizing a positive, slimmer future. Closing their eyes and going forward to next year; seeing themselves at their chosen target weight and size. How do they feel? What do they wear at work? Which shops do they buy their clothes from? Do they still avoid mirrors? How much energy do they have? How confident do they feel? What sorts of things are people saying to them? How has their life changed? Where are they going? What are they going to drink? What are they going to eat? How has being slimmer affected their relationship with their partner? This session is reproduced in Self Hypnosis 1 on page 117.

Session 2

Before attending the clinic for the second session, clients are required to fast from the previous evening. This is in preparation for a blood test which compares cholesterol, triglyceride, and blood-sugar readings at the start of the therapy and then on subsequent visits. This is followed by a test to establish their RMR (Resting Metabolic Rate, described on page 126). This is done using a Korr Metacheck™ device.[1] They are then given an explanation of metabolic rates, calories, portion control, what the body needs and what it doesn't. We look at the role of exercise; we look at 1lb (0.45kg) of fat; and we compare the density of fat and muscle. Then, for the first time, they, and now you, as you read Chapter 7, are faced with the critical question: 'Do you *need* that food, or do you just *want* it?

Hypnosis and Visualization

The session ends with a 20-minute hypnosis session in which clients are asked to picture themselves sitting down to eat a healthy, balanced meal; thinking through the process of producing smaller meals, and serving them on smaller plates; focusing their attention on their food. Eating slowly, and mindfully. Taking smaller mouthfuls. Placing their cutlery on their plate occasionally. Asking themselves if they are really hungry before anything goes in their mouth.

Then they picture themselves at their target weight – focusing their attention on the positive feelings that go with being slim. If they find themselves reaching for food when they're not hungry, their subconscious mind will distract them into doing something else. All of these issues are explored with readers in the next chapter. This hypnosis session is reproduced in Self Hypnosis 2 on page 165.

The client is also introduced to Pause Button Therapy (see Chapter 11).

Session 3

This session focuses on CBT and incorporates a full analysis of all the information obtained during sessions 1 and 2. The client receives explanations as to why they eat and behave in certain ways, and is shown how easily change can be introduced. Techniques are shared that they can use for the rest of their lives.

We also explore the hunger question and define 'fullness'. We look at how we should question everything that we put in our mouths. We ask clients how they got to be the size that they are, and how they maintain their current weight. We calculate how many calories they would need to eat to maintain their current size – they're obviously eating too much and they may have a shock! We ask what their motivation is for losing weight. Does it include health issues along with more emotional aims? We look at wants, needs, desires, cravings; the difference between lapse and relapse; losing weight by 'chunking'; how everything we do starts as a thought. We look at these topics with you in Chapter 8.

Session 4

In this, we review all three previous sessions, going over what clients have learned and achieved so far. How much they can and should eat, and why. What happens once the Gastric Mind Band has been fitted. How the restriction of the Gastric Mind Band will help them reach their target weight and maintain a smaller food intake. We also look at a real surgical gastric band, and watch a film of a banding operation, explaining the operation and its possible side effects.

The session concludes with the actual 'fitting' of the Gastric Mind Band, which is undertaken using deep hypnotherapy and visualization techniques. Professional studio lighting, sound effects and computer-driven vortex aroma devices bring together a 'virtual reality' type experience.

Hypnosis and Visualization

Clients are asked to picture a band being wrapped around the top of their stomach. They clench a golf ball in their hand at the same time as they picture the band being put in place, squeezing tighter as they imagine the band being clicked in its final position. Feeling the golf ball as it signifies their new, smaller stomach capacity; recognizing the restriction on their stomach and being unable to eat as much as before. Being satisfied eating much smaller portions. Eating in response to hunger, rather than for any other reason. Making healthier eating choices. Eating more slowly and mindfully. Recognizing that this is a whole new way of life.

And when they next eat, they notice the difference. This session is reproduced in Self-Hypnosis 3 on page 235.

At the end of the GMB treatment the client is provided with a comprehensive manual, which covers the four sessions in depth. They also receive a set of six CDs, one being a personalized recording of their own sessions, and are given their own complete GMB toolkit to help them adapt to their new lifestyle.

To obtain our dedicated GMB products: the DVD giving more detail of the treatment and containing interviews with clients, or self-hypnosis audio CDs to use for the separate hypnotherapy sessions, visit www.gmband.com

'I've spent thousands of pounds on pills, potions, shakes and liposuction. Now, 11 months on from GMB, I'm over 2 stone (12.7kg) lighter, and not afraid about putting the weight back on.'
GMB CLIENT W. L.

Chapter 6
Session One:
Peeling the Onion

The GMB therapy is not a diet. It's a method of providing the tools you need to achieve a change in your relationship with food, and to show you how you have habitually used food for emotional reasons rather than what it should be used for — fuel.

GMB's a way to understand yourself better — to recognize the choices you've been making, how they've shaped your food shopping, your eating, your body and, ultimately, your life. You can now change those choices, starting today. No, not once you've finished the book, but today, after you've read this chapter! To achieve this, you need to be honest and help build the total picture of why you have a weight problem, why you eat, when you eat, what you eat, and just how often you've been kidding yourself.

If hunger isn't the problem in the first place, then eating will never be the solution.

First, we ask you to read through the questionnaire on the following pages. Then read it again. Then go back and answer the questions. They're designed to help you discover just what your eating habits and patterns are doing to you, and why.

Be honest when you answer the questions – you're not cheating anyone but yourself if you don't give truthful answers. Then *write your answers down* – in a journal, or a notebook, or wherever you wish. They will provide the road map for your personal GMB journey. Knowing your answers – and, especially, seeing them written down – will ensure that, maybe for the first time in your life, you will know more about yourself and the choices and behaviours you most need to address.

Keep this information safe. You may think that once you're on the road to a healthier relationship with food you won't need it any longer. But there are two very good reasons for filing it away. Firstly, so you can go back to it weekly (daily if you need to) and see if you're making the right changes. Secondly, there'll come a time when you realize your life has changed.

When that happens – in the same way that a 'before' photograph is a brilliant incentive to lose weight – a catalogue of your old, bad eating habits will be something to look at and be pleased you've put behind you. It'll remain as a constant mental 'nudge' never to return to those wrong ways.

You may like to ask a close friend or a family member to ask you the questions in the questionnaire – that's ultimately up to you, but never forget that this is *your* journey, no one else's, and you don't need to be judged. You need to make your own decisions for your own reasons. To be successful you have to build what may be a painfully honest picture of your weight history; then, and only then, can you think about addressing change.

Good luck!

The GMB Questionnaire

Session 1 is structured in such a way as to encourage you to ask some pretty heavy, maybe even awkward, questions about yourself, your past and your beliefs. This is designed to prod you and to get you thinking.

It's important that you read and think about the questions in the order in which they're presented – they're in this order for a reason. You should be open and honest with yourself in order to gain the most out of this process.

Before you start, however uncomfortable it is for you, you need to get on the scales and find out how much you weigh now, and make a note of it. You need to know the starting point of your journey. You should also have an idea of the weight you *want* to be, and make a note of this, too. Make a note of your current clothes size, too, and the size that you're aiming to be, but, of course, be realistic. The debate about size zero celebrities and models is contentious for good reason. Don't hanker after the bad flipside of being fat; being underweight is as unhealthy as being overweight.

Those in the medical profession often use a formula called the Body Mass Index (BMI), which is based on the relationship between a person's height and weight, to work out whether they are of normal weight, overweight, or obese. There are other factors worth considering – waist size, body shape, etc. – but as a simple baseline to work from, BMI works for most people.

To work out your BMI you need to know your height in metres and your weight in kilograms (you can use the conversion charts on pages 263–68). Once you've done this, make a note of your current BMI and your desired BMI (a BMI between 18.5 and 24.9 is in the healthy range).

Before you answer any of the questions that follow, you need to get real with yourself. Once you've responded to a question, take another look at your answer, and then go one step deeper inside your head, and your food problems. Then answer the question again, this time even more honestly. It's like peeling an onion. We don't want you to remove just one layer; we want you to peel as deeply as you can, to really expose your reasons for eating to excess on all those occasions.

1. When do you want to reach your target weight/size?

Remember to make your expectations realistic – ideally you should aim to reduce your weight by 1–2lbs (0.45–0.90kg) per week. Grab a calculator and a calendar to find a realistic goal date, and then write it down in your notebook.

2. Is there an outfit in your wardrobe that you'd like to be able to wear again?

Part of the GMB visualization therapy involves you projecting your mind forward in time to when you are your ideal weight and size. Once there, you will picture yourself wearing the outfit in your wardrobe – focusing on how good you're feeling about yourself, proud and confident, slim, attractive, fit, healthy and full of energy.

In psychology this technique is called 'going there first' – athletes regularly use it to picture themselves giving their best possible performance. If you don't have any 'slim' clothes, just think about what sort of outfit you're going to enjoy buying and wearing. How will you look? And, more importantly, how will you feel?

You've only answered two questions so far, but stop right here. If you've got your target date and outfit ready, let's go there right now, in your mind.

Project yourself forward to, let's say, Christmas time. Just for five minutes, sit quietly, alone. Close your eyes and see yourself, *really* see yourself. It's 7 p.m. on Christmas Eve, and you're going out to dinner with your partner and a few friends. You are at your target weight. What will you look like? How much energy and confidence will you have? What fragrance will you be wearing? How will your partner and friends see you and behave towards you? Will your voice be full of pride? Build the picture in your mind.

If you could have that right now – all of it – or a bar of chocolate or a packet of crisps, which would you choose? It's your choice.

Your Childhood and Background

Although we may find it hard to believe and accept, many of our mannerisms, traits, habits, and so on were learned and developed during childhood. Think carefully about your childhood, and then ask yourself if you had any reason to develop issues relating to food and eating as you were growing up. The questions below may help to bring to the surface any possible problem areas.

The more time you spend thinking about these issues the better. Some people have spent two or three days on this section of the questionnaire alone. Take our advice. Go on…

3.   Who brought you up (parents, grandparents, other)?

4.   When you think back, was your childhood happy?

5.   How was your relationship with your family?
Did you feel loved/unloved/wanted/abandoned/lonely/not good enough, etc.?

6.   Were there any problems at home with parents/step-family/siblings?
For example, divorce/separation, etc.?

7.   Was there any abuse – verbal/physical/sexual?

8.   Were there any rivalries in relationships within the home?

9.   Did you have any problems at school – bullying, for example? Did you go to boarding school?

10. How were mealtimes at school?

11. Were you healthy as a child?

12. Were you overweight as a child?

13. How were mealtimes at home?
Were they a pleasant and relaxed family time, or were there rows, stress, etc.?

14. Were you brought up to clear your plate at every meal, and was food ever used as a reward?
For example, did your parents ever say to you that if you clear your plate you can leave the table; if you finish your dinner, you can have an ice cream?

15. Did/do your parents, or any other close family members, have a weight problem?

16. When did your weight first become an issue for you?

17. If you have children, are they overweight?

18. How is your current relationship with your close family?

19. Do you have any problematic relationships in your life at the moment? If so, how do you see them improving?

20. **Do you currently have any problems with your partner, or have you ever experienced problems with previous partners?** Abuse, for example.

21. **Do you or your partner have any children from a previous relationship? If so, are there any problems with those step-children on either side?**

22. **When you think about the questions above – your upbringing, childhood and time at school – what do you remember?**
What were mealtimes like? Were they fun, or stressful? How about school mealtimes? Did your parents encourage you to clean your plate; to eat it all up so you could have some pudding?

23. **How are mealtimes now?**
Are they happy family times or rushed and treated as unimportant events?

Are you peeling the onion? Truly?

The answers to the questions in this section may explain how you came to eat for emotional reasons, rather than hunger. But, realistically, now you have to step well away from that history and create your own healthier new future.

Your Weight History

Take some time now to chart your weight ups and downs over the years – going back to the very first time you were aware of your weight being an issue for you. Include details of any diets that you've followed in the past; note what worked best for you, and what didn't, and why. Think about when you were at your lightest and your heaviest, and how long you stayed at each weight.

Set your notes out along a timeline (draw a straight line on a sheet of paper, then put your birth date at the beginning of the line and the current date at the end of it). Along the rest of the line, mark any significant events – good and bad – and your weight at the time. Then add in any information you can think of that relates exactly to what was going on in your life at that particular time, and how you were feeling. For example, whether you were happy or unhappy, feeling content or lonely, carefree or stressed out, getting married or splitting up, and so on. This should help you realize how different events and emotions have influenced your eating habits over the years.

Maybe you should consider taking a break now. Take some time to allow the information to sink in. You may wish to discuss certain aspects of what you've written, or to check with other family members that your recollection of your childhood is accurate, according to them. You'll be surprised how often your recollections of events differ from those of others.

Your Current Eating Habits

Let's move on to how you eat today.

24. Do you enjoy eating? If yes, why?

This may seem like a funny question, but it's worth asking yourself whether it's the taste, the sensation, the chewing, or the fullness feeling that follows that you enjoy.

People often don't consider these things – if you really do enjoy eating, ask yourself why. Think about it; if you're reading this book it's likely that you have an unhealthy relationship with food. Try to ascertain whether you eat when you're bored, depressed or lonely, and why you've been led to believe that food can overcome these feelings.

25. Do you enjoy cooking? Planning the meal, shopping for the ingredients?

26. How often do you eat out?

27. Do you tend to eat more when eating out?

Are you aware that it's quite common, even for slim people, to eat up to 20 per cent more when compared with eating at home?

28. Who does the food shopping in your household? And who prepares and cooks the food?

29. Who is ultimately responsible for your being overweight?

This is a question that very few people ever really think through, or consider the accurate answer to.

30. Do you eat regularly?

31. Do you eat breakfast?

32. How many meals do you eat per day?

33. Which is usually your main meal of the day?

34. Do you tend to eat quickly?

35. Do you ever find that, when you're eating with a group of people, you're the first to finish?

Overweight people tend to be fast eaters. You should be aware that when your stomach sends hormonal signals to your brain that it's full, it can take up to 20 minutes for the brain to receive the signal, so if you eat too quickly, you'll have already finished your meal before your brain has had a chance to register that you're full, and so you end up feeling uncomfortable because you've eaten too much.[1]

36. Are you constantly thinking about food/the next meal? Do you feel as if your whole life revolves around food?

37. Do you tend to finish everything on your plate? Do you finish off other people's food – your children's, for example?

38. Do you eat large portions at mealtimes?

39. Do you ever feel really stuffed after a meal?

40. Imagine you're sitting down to a meal. Would you eat your favourite thing on the plate first, or save it until last?

This may seem like a strange question, but it's a fact that people with a healthy relationship with food eat their meals in a different order to people who don't. When a slim person sees a meal in front of them, they think, 'I may not get to the end of this meal, and I know that the thing I eat first when I'm hungry I'll enjoy the most, so I'll eat my favourite thing at the front end of the meal. If I'm full before I get to the end, and have to leave something on my plate, it really doesn't matter.'

Most people with an unhealthy relationship with food tend to save the best until last. They use it as a magnet to draw themselves to the end of the meal to ensure they hoover up everything on the plate – whether they're uncomfortably full as they approach the end of the meal or not, they'll always carry on until they've eaten their favourite part.

41. Make a comprehensive list of the types of food you eat, and how frequently.

Here's a sample list: sweets/chocolate biscuits (once a week); cake (twice a month); crisps/savoury snacks (daily); pasta/

rice (three times a week); bread (daily); fruit (once a week); vegetables (twice a day); ready meals (four times a week). Now be honest, and do your own list.

When you really think about it, is it possible that, with just a little more thought, you could make healthier choices when buying and cooking food; choices that would take you closer to your goal, to that place, that time, you pictured a little while ago when you answered the first few questions. That time when you'll feel fitter, healthier and slimmer, and be wearing those clothes you've so longed to wear.

Be honest with yourself: do you think that you eat healthily overall?

42. What are your favourite foods?

43. Which foods do you *not* like?

44. Do you have 'good eating' days and 'bad eating' days? Make a list of what you would eat on a typical 'good eating' day.

Remember to be completely honest with yourself, and include absolutely everything, even the odd snack; also include all drinks. Remember every time you finish off your kids' tea, each nibble you grabbed from the fridge as you walked past it or prepared a meal for someone else.

45. Now make a list for a 'bad eating' day.

46. How often do you have 'bad eating' days? What triggers them?

47. Do you like to finish off a meal with a dessert? Why?

When people in a restaurant order a starter and a main course, the chances of them ordering dessert because they're hungry are remote. They may give in to peer pressure, or be intimidated by the waiter, but they seldom order it because they're hungry.

48. What's your favourite fruit?
It would be far more beneficial for you to start reaching for a refreshing, nutritious piece of fruit than a calorie-dense dessert full of refined sugar.

49. If you're going to snack on something, what will you reach for first?
Think about whether you are a sweet or a savoury person.

50. Do you feel that there's a particular food or food group that's causing your weight problem? And are there any particular foods you would like to cut down on, or cut out altogether?

51. Have you ever given anything up?
For example: sugar/milk/alcohol. Of course, if you have given up something in the past, these small changes you are starting to make will be easy, like a walk in the park.

How's the onion doing?

Real Hunger Versus Desire and Craving

Do you know the difference between hunger, a desire, and a craving to eat?

Hunger: This is a real, physical sensation that can only be experienced if you haven't eaten anything for a good few hours. It's usually signalled by stomach rumblings, low energy, and other symptoms such as irritability or a headache.

Desire: This is just wanting to eat something because you like the look of it. For example, 'fancying' that piece of cake.

Craving: This is usually for something specific – 'I must have some chocolate', or 'I've got to have a McDonald's'.

52. Do you ever eat when you're not hungry?

Think carefully about what your particular triggers are – the things that start you off reaching for food – and make a list of all of them. For instance, do you graze in between meals, constantly picking? Or while you're watching TV? Do you ever eat just to please someone else (when in a restaurant, for example, or as a guest in someone's home, maybe because you don't want to 'offend' them)? Or maybe you eat to distract yourself from something else? Are you a comfort eater – do you eat when you're feeling bored or stressed, happy or sad, celebrating or commiserating, etc.?

53. Do you eat when you're angry or upset?

For example, when you've had a row with someone.

54. Are you a secret eater?

For example, do you eat when everyone else is out of the house? Do you eat something and hide the wrapper; hide the evidence? Or even eat in the car on the way home, and put the packaging in the bin before you see your family?

55. Do you prefer to eat on your own?

56. Do you eat more when you're on your own compared with when you're in the company of others?

For example, would you perhaps order a small green salad when you go out for dinner with friends, and then proceed to empty the contents of the fridge when you get home?

57. Do your slim friends ever say that they can't understand why you're overweight because they never see you eat much?

58. Do you ever get up during the night to eat?

59. How many portions of the following drinks do you consume each day?

- Tea

- Coffee

- Water

- Coca-Cola/other carbonated drinks
  (*Did you realize that a 330ml (11½ oz) can of Coca-Cola contains 140 calories?*)

- Sugar-free drinks
  (*Did you know that after drinking a sweet drink, whether sweetened artificially or with sugar, the body craves more sweetness, and often food? Moreover, the effect is greater with artificial sweeteners.*) [2]

- Fruit juice
  (*Did you know that you should beware the amount of sugar – and therefore calories – in fruit juice, even though it's natural? It's often better to eat the fruit itself instead – that way you get less sugar and more fibre.*)

60. Do you take sugar in your tea/coffee?

61. What sort of milk do you use?

For example, full cream, semi-skimmed, or soya. If you drink tea or coffee with milk or sugar (or even both), grab a calculator and multiply the number you drink each day by 365, and then multiply that by the combined calories in your drinks. You will be amazed by how they mount up, and even more surprised how, by just making one small change, you can achieve a big result.

For example, a person who drinks five cups of tea or coffee a day with semi-skimmed milk consumes 15 calories x 5 cups per day x 365 days in a year: a staggering total of 27,375 calories a year. Of course, if they took a teaspoon (5g) of sugar as well the figure would rise to 54,750 – a weight gain of more than 15lb (6.8kg) a year!

A three-cup-a-day coffee habit, complete with two teaspoons (10g) of sugar for every cup? Simply cutting out the sugar creates an annual deficit of over 35,000 calories. That's a potential weight loss of 10lb (4.5kg).

Your Current Lifestyle

Next, we need to build up a picture, and an understanding, of how you live.

62. Do you enjoy your job?

63. Do you have a lot of stress in your job?

64. How much (number of units) and what type of alcohol do you drink per week?

65. Where and when do you drink alcohol?
(For example, in the evening with a meal, or at the weekend.)

66. Are you concerned about the amount of alcohol you consume?
(In terms of calories consumed/the effect on your health, etc.)

67. How would you feel about reducing your alcohol intake? Would it affect your social life?

68. Do you currently take any exercise? What sort of exercise do you do? For how many hours per week, on average?

69. Do you have any plans to increase the amount of exercise that you do? (Remember, the more you move about, the more calories you'll burn.)

Take another break now, and read this story: it might help you with some of the questions that are coming up.

JAMES'S STORY

James, an old friend of Martin, was taken to hospital with a stroke – he was just 41 years old. It doesn't happen to people that age, does it?

But James was overweight. He was 5ft 7in (1.70m) and weighed around 18 stone (114.5kg). Apparently he'd got up in the night to go to the bathroom and found he'd lost the use of his right arm and leg, and collapsed.

Before the stroke, other than being overweight, James was an all-round good guy. He ran a successful business, had travelled the world, and always enjoyed the high life. He liked to have the best of everything. After the stroke, the use of his arm and leg never returned to any degree where he could manage to look after himself at home – let alone return to his business.

Mentally, it left him with problems too; his memory was unpredictable. After struggling for a few years, he moved to a sheltered housing unit where he now lives alone. His executive car has been replaced by a wine-red mobility scooter; ironic really, considering his favourite tipple had been red wine.

James wishes that someone, anyone, had warned him about the risks he'd been taking. 'If only I could turn back the clock, allowing me to change, put things right, lose weight, cut down on my drinking, take some exercise – anything to get my life back. Of course it'll never happen…'

Living Under a Shadow

At the clinic, we saw a client who'd had a heart attack; luckily he'd made a full recovery. He said the same thing as James: 'If only someone had told me a year, a month, a week or a day before, that it was GOING TO happen, I would have done anything not to live with this fear of it happening again.'

He said that, despite his consultant telling him that he could enjoy a full and normal life, he still lived as if he was disabled. He'd wake in the night having fallen asleep on his arm, and rouse his wife to phone for an ambulance as he thought the numb arm was a symptom of a stroke. Whenever he got indigestion, or started sweating for no apparent reason, he expected the worst. He was only 46, and he and his wife hadn't been abroad on holiday since the heart attack. He preferred to stay close to home because it seemed safer. Of course, any physical manoeuvres in the bedroom were now confined to the couple's memories.

Virtually every day we see people who are overweight but who haven't had a stroke or a heart attack. Neither do they have Type 2 diabetes or colon cancer. Up to that point, they've been lucky. They've got away scot-free. When we see the sadness in their eyes as they recount their stories about the effect their excess weight has had on their lives, we tell them James's story. We explain that, if they take on board the therapy, work with us and shed the excess weight, we can give them their very own 'get out of jail free card' or winning lottery ticket. GMB and PBT will give them the ability to freeze time, and make those changes and new choices in life.

When it comes to entertaining, dining out, and food in general, people's perceptions are often wrong. If you go to a dinner party, are you a guest, or are you a prisoner? Don't say that you *had* to eat all that food. You weren't a prisoner; it's just how you see things. A cop-out, an excuse.

Okay, you've had a break, and read James's tale. On with the questions…

70. What are *your* main reasons for wanting to get slim?
What concerns you the most about being overweight?

Write down five reasons in your notebook. Really take your time to answer this question. Think of your onion-peeling, because you'll be using these reasons as part of a powerful motivational technique.

Once you've written down the five things that are most important to you, you should regard your list as a sort of contract with yourself – this is what you want to achieve and why. It's much more effective when you put something in writing, rather than just thinking about it and then pushing it to the back of your mind again.

You can then keep a copy of your reasons somewhere handy, so you can whip them out and instantly refresh your memory about exactly where you're aiming to get to, whenever you're in a situation where you're feeling tempted to eat something that you don't need. Use your reasons to decipher what's more important to you – the short-term, instant gratification of eating, or the long-term benefits of getting slim.

How Do You Feel About Being Overweight?

71. Has being overweight affected your self-confidence?

72. Do you feel that your weight has an effect on your relationship with your partner? If yes – how?

73. Do you enjoy being overweight?

74. If you think in terms of a cost-benefit analysis, can you think of any downsides to changing your habits?

For example, you may have to find something other than eating to relieve boredom – you won't be able to give yourself the excuse that you're upset and want a bar of chocolate. This is going to require a certain amount of effort on your part, rather than continuing as you are now. What downsides can you find? And how will you deal with them? Write them down.

75. Can you think of any benefits to maintaining your current weight?

For example, maybe your weight has been a protective shield from any unwanted attention.

76. How certain are you – on a scale of 1–10 – that you want to make the change?

Hopefully you're at a definite 10, and the pros of shifting your excess weight will outdo the cons of staying the way you are. Give yourself some time to think about this. Where are you on the scale?

77. Again, using a scale of 1–10, how *confident* are you that you can make these changes?

Think about what you've achieved in the past when you've put your mind to something. A school sports day win? A good grade in an exam? Passing your driving test? Anything so important to you that you put your mind to it, made an effort and achieved what you wanted. You should approach GMB with the same attitude. Remember, even small changes will add up to a big result in the end. So, how confident are you now that you can make changes?

Making the Commitment

Now we're going to take a look at your innermost feelings about your weight – the often negative effect it has had on your confidence, and the part it plays in your relationship with your partner or other family members. While some of the questions that follow may seem strange, you should spend a considerable amount of time thinking them through, and considering how the answer to one question affects your thoughts on the next.

78. **Are you concerned about your health, and the implications of your weight, not only on yourself, but on your family and loved ones?**

79. **Are you happy with your life?**

80. **Do you consider that you have a lot of stress in your life?**

81. **If you could change one thing in your life, right here, right now, other than your weight, what would it be?**
Stop and think for a moment. This question is probably one of the most important of all. You cannot spend too much time thinking about and analysing the answer you give.

82. **How long do you want to live for? Why?**

83. **Are you afraid of dying?**

84. Who is important to you?

85. Who are you important to?

86. Are you committed to losing weight?

87. What is stopping you?

The use of fear in therapy seldom helps achieve permanent change; however, we want you to be aware that the risk of Type 2 diabetes, stroke and certain cancers goes hand in hand with obesity. Maybe James's story will serve as that particular wake-up call. (Go back and read it again if you're in any doubt.)

When you talk about the risks, the pain and the desperation that many people go through regarding their weight, you ask them whether the burger or whatever is really worth all that; can they really think it's *that* good? Weight loss is not rocket science. It's not expensive, it's not painful, its benefits can last a lifetime, and virtually everyone can achieve it.

88. Are you prepared to accept the consequences of your actions?

The final question perhaps sums it all up: are you prepared to accept the consequences of your actions in life? If you are, and you are ready to make a few – some only temporary – changes, then really there is no reason why your journey can't start right here, right now.

Learn to hold yourself accountable
for all your actions.

Face to face, in the clinic, it would take around four hours to harvest the information we need. You're reading the questions from the book, so you're not talking to someone, hearing their responses, getting feedback, having the question reflected back in a different way, and so on. However, as you complete the questionnaire on your own, it's important to be thorough and completely honest, thinking back to your childhood where appropriate because, as we said earlier, many issues, bad habits and the seeds of distorted thinking often stem from that time in our lives.

Once you think you've finished, go back and check your answers. Make sure you've been honest. Change anything you think you need to. How could the issues the questions raise have affected your eating habits? Your behaviour around food?

The Fork in the Road

If you've decided that your answers are accurate, you're now in a position to move on. This is the time to starting looking ahead; no more looking over your shoulder at the past. Here and now, at this very moment, you're at a crossroads in your life. You've obviously had enough of being overweight, feeling frumpy, unhealthy, struggling to climb stairs, being fed up with your limited choice of clothes. Feeling embarrassed in front of your husband/wife/children's friends. Feeling depressed at the very sight of a mirror. You've got to the decision point. It's crunch time.

You don't need reminding that you did this to yourself, but you're open to suggestions as to how to change. You've probably admitted by now that there's something wrong which dieting hasn't sorted out. You needed to bring forgotten things to the surface. That's why honesty is so important when completing the questionnaire. If you've been saying that you live on salads but are actually a burger-and-fries junkie, it won't help you one bit, because you'll end up completely off track.

Look at yourself as if through someone else's eyes. How much excess weight are you carrying? What would you advise? What would you do? What would you think of that person? What would you say if it were your brother, your sister, or your best friend? If you're upset by these thoughts, that's not unusual. But you need to see yourself as others see you, because in these four sessions what we're trying to do is get you to the right place for you (not us) to bring about change.

We don't want to be judgemental — you've probably spent enough time putting yourself down, so you don't need any more of that. You need to decide that you've got to the end of all the negativity, begin to feel better about yourself and put a positive twist on things.

Say to yourself: 'Right, that's it. I'm sick of it.
I want something different now. It's crunch time.
I'm not playing the victim for a day longer.'

So, you're at a fork in the road of your life. Will you decide to keep heading down that same old road? It's the easiest thing in the world to do; you wouldn't need to make any effort at all. It's a well-trodden route — the path of least resistance. It's up to you.

Stand at that fork now, and think what you'd feel like a year from now if nothing changes. If you carry on doing exactly what you're doing. It would be another year of being overweight, feeling bad about yourself, comfort eating, looking older, feeling terrible, getting out of breath. If nothing changes in your life, just how fat will you be this time next year? Don't be under the illusion that you'll be the same as you are now, because you won't. It'll be worse. It always is. Maybe much worse.

But, to feel like that for another year is not why you're reading this book. Take yourself back to that fork and have a look at how different it's going to feel if you take the *other* road. Make a little bit of an effort; make a few changes. So, a year ahead on this road, you can see all the positive things – you're lighter than you were a year ago, you're fitter, you feel healthy, you don't get out of breath any more.

You look in the mirror and you look a lot younger. You have so much energy; your clothes fit you; you are feeling good about yourself. If you have a partner, they're looking at you admiringly. Everything's great in your family, in your relationships; everything's so much better. There are lots of positive things to focus on.

If you think calmly and deeply enough about the two options – another year as you are versus the positive, vibrant new year after making a few changes – you might find yourself getting quite upset at the thought of how things have been and how they *could* be.

Maybe you doubt you can make the change? And what about the costs? Well, financially they're probably close to zero. Physically, it won't resemble having hot pins poked in your eye. You know it won't hurt. It may feel strange for a little while because you're changing those old habits, but eventually it will become the norm.

Changing Your Behaviour

In fact, with regard to change, we all go through it in much the same way. There's actually an academic theory called the 'Stages of Change Model', which says that everyone makes changes in their life in essentially the same pattern, but taking vastly different times to do so. It's not unusual, in fact its quite normal, to start doubting you even need to change!

The Stages of Change pattern of behaviour change is as follows.[3]

1. **Pre-Contemplation.** At this stage a person has not yet acknowledged that a problem exists, or that there's a problem that needs addressing.

2. **Contemplation.** Now the person recognizes that there's a problem, but is often not yet clear as to whether they want to/know how to make a change.

3. **Preparation/Determination.** Now the person is preparing to make a change.

4. **Action/Willpower.** At this point, change in behaviour is being introduced/practised.

5. **Maintenance.** Keeping up the new behaviours that are the focus of the change.

6. **Relapse.** This is when a person returns to their old behaviours, bringing about a sense of failure. However, it is possible for you to use this as a learning tool – just as we are trying to teach you to do – understanding why you went wrong and how not to 'fail' again as you continue your change.

Or, put more simply:

1. You don't even realize there's a problem.

2. You know there's a problem but you aren't sure what, if anything, to do about it.

3. You know what to do and are starting to do it.

4. You've learned to make the changes and are living with them consistently.

5. You slip and return to old behaviours, but, despite a sense of failure, you now know how to learn from that and get back to changing.

All of this will sound quite familiar to many overweight people who have shed excess weight in the past. Often you get through one or two parts of the sequence, only to slip and go back into an earlier stage, and then get swept into a cycle. Everyone's cycle goes at a different rate – maybe passing through different stages a varying number of times – and overweight people trying to lose weight will see this as a vicious circle rather than something they have to go through before they'll achieve what they want.

'Don't fear failure. Learn from it. See it as an education.'
Martin Shirran

Some people think there's a final part of the pattern – Transcendence – in which you are 'past' the change process and making that lifelong commitment to permanent change. We are confident that with the Gastric Mind Band therapy this is exactly what you'll achieve.

So. You're ready. You're prepared to make that little bit of effort, make those changes, because even a few months down the line, you'll know it's so worth it.

And for some of you, the changes will be at least as much about your health as about your clothes size. About avoiding diabetes, a heart attack and a stroke as much as about how you feel in your swimwear on the beach.

Younger people tend not to prioritize these health concerns and think more about their appearance. Once you're a parent of teenagers, though, your thoughts run to, 'Can I keep up with them when they play football on the beach?', or 'Will I live long enough to see them get married/have my grandchildren?' and 'Will I be healthy enough to enjoy my retirement (if I get there)?' and all the other associated health fears of mid-life.

THE TOP TEN REASONS CLIENTS VISIT THE CLINIC

1. The fear of discovering that the aircraft seat belt is not large enough to go around your stomach, and having to ask for an extension. Followed by the worst nightmare of all – crew using the call button to attract the attention of a steward at the back of the plane, and calling down the aircraft, 'An extension seat belt please for seat 6A.'

2. The total, utter embarrassment and shame of being pleaded to by your daughter or son not to walk them to school any more because the other children in the playground poke fun at them because of your size.

3. Chafing legs; being utterly fed up with having sore thighs caused by them rubbing together when you walk.

4. Having returned from yet another horrid family holiday where you were uncomfortable on the beach, spending the whole time trying to cover up the rolls of fat.

5. Wanting to go to a restaurant and not be aware that everyone else is watching what you order and what you eat.

6. Sick of not being able to bend over to cut your own toenails.

7. Noticing that on the plane, the empty (or half empty) seat next to you was the only one not taken. This was after the steward had asked you when you boarded if you were pregnant – you weren't of course, but at least it would have been an excuse.

8. Realizing that your bathroom scales no longer go up to your weight.

9. To be able to have a bath – that is, to fit in it – and be able to get out afterwards without thinking you may have to ask for assistance.

10. Just once, to be in the wonderful position where you can go to a so-called 'normal' clothes shop, rather than having to buy your clothes from the XXL catalogue.

A Reality Check

When we think of the people reading this book, we think of the clients we've seen sitting in front of us at the clinic, all in exactly the same place in their life. Yes, they may be morbidly obese, and yes, they may have some illusion that being slim will make them feel more attractive and save their marriage. But in reality, what we actually see is someone who's quite young but could be about to have a stroke, resulting in them not being able to go to the bathroom on their own any more because they can't clean themselves.

We see the downsides. If you think about having Type 2 diabetes, and maybe losing the sight in one eye, maybe both, or losing a limb... if you think about them long and hard, we want to ask: 'Do you really still want that pork pie?'

That's the fork in the road you're at, right here, right now. The pork pie and all the downsides of obesity, or to be slim and healthy next Christmas?

Check the health risks out for yourself. Google them. It's not an unrealistic scenario: it's very, very real. The connection between Type 2 diabetes and obesity is off the scale – it's similar to the connection between smoking and lung cancer but, until recently, diabetes hasn't had quite the same level of publicity.

If you carry on eating like you have been until now, getting fatter and fatter, you may find yourself getting closer to Type 2 diabetes, which many now say is developing into a disease of choice.

Small Changes Lead to Big Results

People – we, you, all of us – have 'stuff', or emotional baggage. Sometimes it takes a while just to peel away the layers of the onion. Stuff like, 'I eat because my husband won't talk to me'.

With some people, it's obvious that their weight problem stems from their childhood – perhaps they were always told to clear their plate, whether they were hungry or not. Maybe food was scarce because of lack of money, or perhaps it was of poor quality and had to be eaten up. With others, there are more deep-seated psychological issues: it can be a build-up of various things that have happened in their lives. But there's usually a trigger – it's rare for there to be nothing.

With others still, it's just a change of lifestyle. Perhaps they've gone from working full-time, running around after people, bringing up children, being active and fit, to suddenly retiring and doing nothing, without reducing the amount of food they're consuming. Or they've moved home, or suddenly have more time on their hands.

For some women, it's only when they hit the menopause that they start to have problems. At this time their bodies can build up insulin resistance, and have difficulty processing refined carbohydrates. Because the carbs don't get absorbed properly, the body just takes all the calories from them and these can turn to fat. This can lead to Type 2 diabetes, which means that menopausal women have to watch their intake of refined carbs.[4]

Very often, people who are overweight eat quickly; some 90 per cent of overweight people who come through our doors admit to eating too fast. When you eat quickly, you can consume more food than if you eat slowly, because by the time your brain gets the message that you're full, it's too late – you've stuffed everything into your mouth already. However, even a simple change, like slowing down and eating mindfully rather than just shovelling everything in mindlessly and not paying attention to what you're eating, can have a big effect.

A lot of the GMB therapy is about every small change developing into a larger, cumulative effect. You don't have to make huge changes in everything.

SLOW DOWN YOUR EATING

In order to get the most from food you love, it should stay in your mouth – where your taste receptors are – for as long as possible. You won't get the most from it if it's already down your throat and on its way to your stomach.

Try staying in the moment: enjoy the taste, the texture, the smell and the appearance of what you are eating.

To help you learn to eat more slowly, we recommend that you start by swapping cutlery hands for a week. Then, just when you've got the hang of that, switch to chopsticks – even when you're eating baked beans on toast! The following week, revert to normal – you'll find you're already eating more slowly. The fact that you've had to keep sweeping up the mess from eating in an unfamiliar way will have created some 'non-eating' time, too – plus you will burn some extra calories!

By concentrating on eating more slowly, you'll move yourself down the path of creating a better and more mindful eating habit.

One of our clients didn't seem to overeat that much, but she liked to have a couple of vodka and Cokes when she got home from work. We showed her how these contributed 84,000 extra calories to her intake every year, and that just by cutting them out, it could mean a weight loss of over 24lb (10.9kg) over 12 months with no other changes. Just cutting out those drinks. Guaranteed. Did she need us to tell her that? Small change = very big result.

Do You Eat Mindfully or Mindlessly?

Do you think about the colour or texture of your food? Or where it's come from or what processes it's gone through? Does this mean you're eating *mindfully* or *mindlessly*? Do you analyse the tastes and textures of the food in your mouth as you're chewing it? You only have taste buds in your mouth, not your stomach, so the longer the food stays in your mouth, the more pleasure you obtain from it.

As you start to eat more mindfully, you can almost feel as though your palate is changing. Gradually, you'll realize that healthy food actually tastes a whole lot better than unhealthy food. If you take a bite of a big sticky bun and eat it slowly – so it spends a lot of time in your mouth – you'll start to notice all the fat coating your tongue and sticking to the roof of your mouth, and the amount of sugar you can taste. You'll realize there's little, if any, texture. It may take a while, but your tastes will gradually turn away from what we call 'beige' foods – the high-carbohydrate junk that is stuffed full of 'empty' calories and has very poor nutritional value.

Staying on the theme of colour, it's quite widely believed that one of the easier ways to ensure you have a healthy diet is to eat as many different-coloured foods in any meal as you possibly can (not counting multi-coloured cereals or sweets of course!). US writer Michael Pollan has highlighted the theory that it's not wise to eat any breakfast cereal that colours the milk[5] – sensible advice if you stop and think about it.

Do you eat regular, proper meals, or just graze continually? Maybe you're almost frightened of feeling hunger and pick at bits and pieces all day long because hunger feels like a life-or-death situation? Perhaps you think that it's not good to feel hungry, so you just keep on eating. You never get empty, never get hunger pangs, and are therefore completely out of touch with your body's natural signals.

Constantly eating also means that the stomach never gets thoroughly emptied; it may even stretch over time, so you need to eat more before you feel satisfied.

Some diets actually promote the idea that feeling hungry is a negative thing, and even go as far as stating, 'if you follow this diet you'll never feel hungry'. We don't like that idea. Hunger pangs are a natural, positive sensation. They are simply your body's way of letting you know that it's time to eat something. They aren't a brush with death! If somebody is eating and it's not a response to hunger, that's an emotional issue; eating for head hunger rather than stomach hunger. Learn to live with, and accept, hunger and you'll learn to live more comfortably with food.

Instead of fearing hunger, try tolerating it!

Once you start to understand the notion of real hunger, you'll also realize there are different 'grades' of hunger. If you fancy an apple, is that hunger or are you making excuses? Well, yes, it is hunger, but it's obviously not full-blown 'I need a meal' hunger. If you eat a piece of fruit, it should really be enough to tide you over for another couple of hours or so, until you need a meal.

Sometimes people like to have fruit – maybe several pieces – during the day. Is that fulfilling hunger for a little while or eating too often? We believe there's no harm at all in having a piece of fruit or a yoghurt or something, but *only* if you're feeling hungry. It's important to be careful with fruit, too – it's delivered to your mouth complete with its own natural sugars.

It's a little known fact that you can eat too much fruit![6] When you eat other sugars, insulin is released, which means the brain knows when you've had enough to eat. So high insulin levels quell appetite. Fruit contains fructose, though, which doesn't stimulate insulin or leptin – the hormone that makes you feel full – so, in theory, you could eat excessive quantities of fruit without ever feeling satisfied.

Some people can go longer than others without eating. Those who are cutting down noticeably on their portion sizes might find that after two, three, four hours, they need a little something, but not everyone does. Some people will just have their meals and not need anything in between at all. Don't eat just for the sake of it: eat if you're feeling a bit peckish.

If you allow yourself to get completely ravenous, you're more likely to eat too quickly, and be tempted to overeat. It's better to have a piece (one piece!) of fruit, or something small, every so often, because each time you eat your metabolism kicks in. You shouldn't go for more than about five or six hours without a little something to eat. After this amount of time, your body starts shutting down, going into starvation mode – inhibiting calorie burn and slowing your metabolic rate.

Are You an Emotional Eater?

What would you think if a friend of yours was drinking a bottle of cough mixture every day to overcome sore feet caused by tight shoes? You'd probably think it was strange, weird even?

Or if another friend told you they're taking laxatives on a daily basis to ease their toothache? If an overweight friend told you that they eat a family-sized bar of chocolate before bed every night to take away their loneliness, would you think this was stranger still?

Is taking cough mixture for aching feet really any more peculiar, or less believable, than someone eating chocolate – or cheese sandwiches – in the evening because they're lonely? Sadness, being lonely, and feeling anxious are emotions. Signals to change something in your life. They are *never* an instruction to eat.

People with an unhealthy relationship with food seldom eat excessively because they're hungry. It's amazing how many of them eat because they are feeling depressed, lonely or tired – they have a distorted view that such feelings and emotions can somehow, as if by magic, be overcome by food.

Say you've had a row with your best friend. What do you do? Go and have a bar of chocolate – *that'll* make you feel better. But how do you feel afterwards? Still upset with your friend. And even more upset with yourself for eating the chocolate.

What would have been more helpful? Did the chocolate actually help? No, it didn't – you were feeling upset *before* you ate it, and then after it'd gone, you felt bad about yourself because you'd eaten chocolate you didn't need. All you really needed to do was have a good cry, pick up the phone, apologize to your friend, sort it out with her and forget the chocolate. How was eating chocolate a logical thing to do?

Once you learn to use your Pause Button (coming up in Chapter 11) when you feel like picking up a chocolate bar, you'll give yourself time to see how much more angry, upset and depressed you'll feel after eating it, and give yourself the time to opt out of unwrapping it – way before you get close to biting into it.

Hopefully, by now you'll have been laughing at yourself – seeing all the places where you've been going wrong. The chocolate (or whatever you reached for) only comforts you temporarily, for the few minutes or seconds it takes you to eat it. The feel-good factor doesn't balance out the guilt afterwards; the beating yourself up about it because you didn't need it anyway. Now you've stuffed up your diet and you're feeling bad about yourself, so you're going to eat even more, you're likely to put weight on and therefore get into that whole negative cycle.

Maybe your problem is dealing with 'bored' moments? Well, there's always something you could do instead of eating when you feel bored. What do you enjoy: reading, working on the computer? You could walk around the block; email some friends; investigate a new hobby. There are plenty of things to occupy your time other than using food as an emotional crutch.

Food doesn't solve anything other than satisfying your body when it's hungry: eating doesn't overcome emotions.

If you enjoy a meal with friends, the food is really only the catalyst for spending time with people you like; something to do while you chat, laugh, joke, and so on. In great company you could take an hour to eat one plate of salad and have a better time than you would eating a heavy three-course meal with boring people and experiencing that guilt trip later.

THE DEMON DRINK (NUTRITIONALLY SPEAKING!)

If you drink alcohol – even a little – it may play a far greater part in your weight problem than you realize because it's easy to overlook the calories you're consuming. On top of that, the body can't store alcohol at all, so it has to process it, even before processing food. So, if you're having food *and* alcohol, it'll metabolize the alcohol first, get all the calories that way, and if your body's reached its calorie requirement for the day, the food won't get processed properly and will be stored as fat.

Alcohol also increases appetite, so once you start drinking, you're also likely to eat more food.[7] All of which isn't a problem if it's under control. Also, if you're at your normal weight, you can afford to consume more calories than someone who's overweight because if you're trying to lose weight you have to create a deficit. Someone at normal weight is just eating to maintain their weight as it is. There's one additional problem with alcohol – it can *reduce* a person's metabolic rate – a frightening thought![8]

Low Frustration Tolerance

There's a pattern called Low Frustration Tolerance (LFT). Whether it's drugs, alcohol, food, or gambling, it's said that the person has LFT to that particular issue.[9] They get a craving to have a cigarette, or go to the betting shop, or have a doughnut, and as soon as they have that thought, they respond to it immediately because they see it as a command which has to be obeyed. They can't work their way through this craving – it's their LFT to that particular thing. They may have a high tolerance for all other things in their lives – for an overweight person it may be that they'd never touch cigarettes because they're bad for your health and taste and smell horrible – but food cravings are what they have LFT to.

If you see a food advertisement, would you get up and have something to eat, even if you'd just had dinner? One person can handle a particular LFT better than another. Marion would not give in to a doner kebab at lunchtime, whereas Martin would have done, though not any longer!

The first technique for overcoming LFT is to recognize what it is. For you, it may be that you're eating salad but giving in to having some bread that you didn't really need but automatically picked up. Or it may be that you simply took a sweet that was offered to you without thinking.

Stress and boredom often play a part. When stressed, a slim person probably can't eat, whereas a stressed overweight person will eat constantly. And if a stressed overweight person eats, it's because, for whatever psychological reason, they're thinking that the food is going to help them feel better. Once you develop a habit like this, it becomes so strongly ingrained in your mind that it comes naturally, and you'll do it automatically, without even thinking about it. Eating too much is a habit. But habits can be broken!

The easiest thing in the world is to keep on doing what you've been doing. To actually make the changes – create new habits – requires a bit of effort, which in turn requires motivation. But once you've done something – made new choices, thought in different ways – a few times, it gets easier and easier.

You can learn if you want to. If you've always driven on the left and you suddenly have to drive on the right, you can do it, even if you doubt yourself and your ability to unlearn your existing habit. You have to concentrate the first few times, but after a while it becomes second nature.

Identifying Your Motivations for Losing Weight

The following list of suggestions may help you identify your main motivations for shifting your excess weight, but if they're not for you, you can come up with your own list.

- I want to *feel* healthier and I want to *be* healthier.

- I want to look better for me.

- I want to be more attractive for my partner.

- I want to feel more confident.

- I want to be able to walk into a 'normal' clothes shop and buy things easily, knowing they'll fit.

- I want to be able to buy things that I like rather than just because they're the only things in the shop that will fit me. No more zero choice.

- I want to have more energy.

- I don't want to get breathless walking up stairs, or to the bus stop.

- I want to be a better role model for my children.

- I don't want to end up like my family member who died at an early age.

- I want to be able to live my life and enjoy it, rather than just existing.

- I want to feel normal rather than the 'fat person in the room'.

- I don't enjoy socializing because of how I feel, and I want to have an active social life once more.

- I've had enough of yo-yo dieting.

- I want to pay 'normal' prices for clothes, rather than having to buy expensive outsized items.

- I don't want to feel like the 'Michelin man', with these spare tyres always with me.

- I want to be active again.

- I want to feel in control of food, rather than controlled by it.

- I don't want to always worry about what people think about my eating.

- I want to be able to join in with my kids' activities.

So, what have you identified as your most important motivation? Is it your health? To change your shape before the next 'big' birthday, or just to feel better about yourself? Everyone's will be different, or in a different order, but what matters is yours and yours alone – and *it* will be *your* motivation.

Note your motivations in your notebook or diary, save them to your iPhone, create a new screensaver; or just make sure you keep them in your handbag or wallet. Then, if you're tempted by a bar of chocolate, or if you're about to sit down to a meal, whip them out, and read them to remind yourself of them. You can even read through them at the start of each new day.

Your list will remind you that this is what's important to you right now, and that you want to be able to do this because…

Making a note of your motivations, something to read, makes an amazing difference. It's like making a commitment – almost a 'legally binding document' with yourself. It's helpful, and it really works. Keep the list handy so you can keep reinforcing all these positive things. If you've got a cream cake in one hand and the reasons *not* to eat it in the other, press Pause, and give yourself time to think (see Chapter 11).

THE IMPORTANCE OF FUTURE THINKING

It is really useful to identify and remind yourself frequently of your future goals in terms of weight loss. According to the theory of Time Perspective, developed by Prof Philip Zimbardo, people separate into three basic types:

Past Thinkers, whose lives and decision-making are dominated by events in the past;

Present Thinkers, who seek immediate gratification, and are often influenced by physical sensations such as hunger or thirst. They rarely plan ahead.

Future Thinkers are aware of the consequences of their actions, plan well ahead and are often conscientious and controlled.

Altering your thinking to learn a new, more normal relationship with food as a fuel requires that you understand that today's eating affects tomorrow's weight (or next week's, next year's or even your weight a decade away)… which of course if you've had a weight problem, is not at the forefront of your mind when faced with one of your 'trigger' foods or smells.

You have to learn to alter your Present Thinking to take account of Future Consequences, by identifying and prioritizing the Motivations you've just listed.

What's more important: a quick sugar fix which will last five minutes maximum, and then you'll feel bad about yourself for the rest of the day because you didn't actually need it, or the long-term benefits of shedding your excess weight?[10] You decide.

Each time you're about to take a mouthful of food, stop and think. Ask yourself: 'Is this going to help me achieve what I want, or hinder me?' If you're hungry, it's going to help. Go ahead and eat it. But if you're not, and it's going to hinder your progress, why on earth would you be doing it?

Ask yourself: 'Will this piece of cheese, packet of crisps or doughnut help me slim down to 10 stone (63.6kg); will it help me move closer or further away from my goal? Which do I want more? If

I want the food more, I can go ahead. But if the most important thing in my life is to slim down, why am I making it harder for myself by still eating the wrong things that aren't going to help me achieve that?'

No one is actually holding you down and forcing all that extra food into your mouth. You can choose to keep on eating too much, or you can choose to be slimmer and healthier. Realistically, you can't have both, so make your choice.

Diet Is a Dirty Word

Diets tend to mess you up mentally, and make you more obsessed with food than you were before. It's only when you deal with the underlying issues around your relationship with food – the ones that you identified in the questionnaire – that you'll be able to make a permanent change.

Don't put your life on hold. You have to get out of the dieting mentality. If you're going out, you need to behave differently when you're making food and drink choices. You have to lead a normal life, have normal social engagements, without the 'I'm on a diet so I can't do anything' way of thinking.

From now on you should be asking yourself the following question every time you're about to eat: 'Am I eating this because I'm actually hungry?' If, instead, it's because you're bored, sad, lonely, or stressed, or because you've had a row with your boss, put it down!

You must question every food choice during the first few days and weeks, until you get into the new pattern/routine. Food choice = Pause Button moment! To live like a slim person lives for life, you've got to develop a good relationship with food. There's nothing wrong with enjoying your food. Why on earth would you make it a torturous process when you could make it something that's really pleasurable? You could enjoy eating things that make you feel fit and healthy rather than sluggish.

> *'A diet isn't something you do for life, it's some kind of purgatory you go through for a certain number of weeks, and then heave a big sigh of relief as you go back to the "normal" eating habits that made you overweight in the first place.'*
> **MARION SHIRRAN**

Of course, the quicker you eat, the less you'll actually taste your food. Conversely, the longer the food stays in your mouth, the more you'll realize the taste of it and maybe reduce your desire for it. Cake and biscuits? There's a good chance you'll decide that, actually, they don't taste that nice after all and you'd rather have an apple! People do have these light-bulb moments, because with typical comfort food, they haven't been eating for the flavour, they've been eating for the effect. Soothing ice cream, melt-in-the-mouth chocolate... they are nothing more than a quick sugar fix. It's no coincidence that comfort food is like baby food: stodgy, mushy stuff.

For encouragement, keep a 'before' photo stored away with your completed questionnaire. Then, maybe not that many weeks down the line, you can get another picture taken – make sure you are wearing the same clothes so you can see the difference as your weight changes – and be aware of the benefits as they happen.

It helps to have an idea of your ups and downs, too – how long you've stayed at a particular weight, then put it on again, lost it again. Do you sometimes avoid the scales? That's burying your head in the sand, and you'll probably end up putting on more weight than you think. When you're in control, and you weigh yourself regularly (say monthly), you'd never allow that to happen.

Think of the process not as 'losing' weight, but as gaining a better life.

Don't make the mistake of expecting too much too soon. You may well lose weight easily and quickly from the very start – many people do – but don't set an unrealistic target and an unrealistic deadline. It might have taken you years to become this overweight, so you can't expect to lose it in a couple of weeks.

If you've got a lot of weight to lose, your initial target may still be within the overweight range, but what matters is that for you, it'll be the lightest you've been for a long time (or ever). Once you're there, you can reassess if you want to keep going, or are happy at that weight. For somebody who's never been slim, it can be difficult to imagine being within the normal parameters of the BMI.

Did you work out your BMI earlier? Is it outside the normal range? Well, let's be clear. Telling you in no uncertain terms that you should reduce your BMI is not so much a proverbial kick up the backside as much as letting you know you're at high risk for Type 2 diabetes, coronary heart disease and colon cancer (to name just three obesity-related conditions). Please focus on whether you want a burger, along with diabetes, or whether you'd rather have a piece of grilled fish and be slim by your next birthday. It's your choice, of course. The questionable pleasures of the burger will last five minutes or so; the associated diabetes could be with you for life. What's your decision?

'This was one of the most profound experiences of my life. It changed my perceptions about myself inside and out: about food, my body, my mind, the untapped power we have at our fingertips that we are unaware of. I gained self-confidence and self-respect, and a more positive outlook on my life.'

US GMB CLIENT

Taking Your Measurements

We always suggest that you measure your problem spots – maybe your hips, waist, bust, tops of arms and legs – every couple of weeks. It's up to you which bits you measure, but it's probably best that they are where you're most looking forward to seeing the numbers go down! If you start taking more exercise, you may not see your weight dropping because of the different density of muscle and fat. Knowing that your body *is* changing, even if your weight has plateaued out, is a valuable lesson that can stop you from getting disillusioned, and keep you on track. Measurements can be as important as scales!

According to a British survey taken in 1951, the average woman's waist size was 70cm (27.5in). In 2011 it was 76.2cm (30in.)[11] Another way to determine obesity is by using the waist–hip ratio. Divide your waist measurement by your hip measurement. The ideal ratio, around 0.8 for women and 0.95 for men, is a strong indicator of general health.[12]

MARION SHIRRAN'S STORY

Marion has been slim all her life. Because of her professional training, and years spent in conversation with overweight people – hearing their thought processes, fears and doubts – she understands only too well how the whole process of weight loss can become obsessive.

A fussy eater as a child, Marion was brought up with home-cooked meals, home-grown vegetables, and a very patient and laid-back Mum who let her and her sister eat as little as they wanted, knowing they'd eventually come back for more if they got hungry.

Though her tastes broadened considerably as she grew up, Marion admits to still loving some of her childhood preferences – fish-finger sandwiches, milky puddings, and mashed banana.

Now a keen cook, and still a fan of chocolate, cheese and cream – three of the 'nightmare' foods for the weight-obsessed – Marion's mindset is clear, and clearly very different from that of those who eat too much.

Marion's philosophy is: 'Food is a fuel. Eat what you want, but *only* if you're hungry. Only eat until you're satisfied – and not too fast, or you'll trick your brain.' It's a simple message, and it's hard to tease any more out of her because the fact is, that's how she thinks. If she walked past a fruit bowl, would she eat a banana if it looked good? Not a chance… unless she was hungry.

Would she sneak a plate of cold rice pudding from the fridge just because it's her favourite? No, not unless she was hungry. She can't give any more explanation than that, because it's straightforward. Why would you eat if you're not hungry? Why would you eat food on a plate if you don't like it? Why would you eat food even if you *do* like it, if you're already full?

'I eat an extremely varied diet,' Marion explains. I don't have any forbidden foods because I eat everything in moderation.'

GMB as a Way of Life

Now in her mid-40s, Marion wears the same clothes size as she did in her teens.

'Many of our clients take one look at me and say that I'm lucky because I don't have a weight problem. They're envious, and say things like, "I bet you can eat whatever you like and never put on weight." I suppose that's true – I can and do eat whatever I like – but I guess the difference between them and me is that I wouldn't dream of overeating, or eating when I'm not hungry. So, I wouldn't class myself as lucky that I stay slim; it's simply because I do eat whatever I want to, but I only eat when I physically need to.

'Martin and I do drink alcohol, but usually only at weekends, and we'll enjoy a few glasses of wine every day while on holiday.

'A number of clients have said that if someone could come up with a pill to take daily instead of having to eat food, they'd be happy to take it because the whole stressful business of eating would be gone forever. I feel sad that they have such a strained relationship with food that they've lost the art of enjoying eating.'

In fact, Marion's an advocate of 'real' food – she would choose butter over margarine any day for its taste, and because it's not processed. She'd opt for a regular coffee rather than decaffeinated. She wonders why people choose low-fat foods, because sugar has been added to them to enhance their taste.

So, does her weight fluctuate? In some circumstances – for example, if she's on a cruise, where the diet is much richer than normal – she acknowledges that her weight can go up. But when it does, she's on top of it very rapidly. 'You can tell by your clothes if you're altering at all,' she says. 'My weight never varies by more than five or six pounds (2.26–2.72kg) at most – it's that much up or down and that's it.

People who've been on diets become absolutely obsessed with the scales, weighing themselves every time they go to the bathroom. For me to try and get inside their heads, I've experimented and weighed myself several times a day and seen that my weight fluctuates by a huge amount. From morning to evening I can put on 3lb (1.35kg). It's not that I've actually put on weight: it's just the food and liquid I've consumed gradually working its way through my digestive system.

'But people get so worked up about that with the whole dieting mentality. They'll see their weight creeping up during the day, and that makes them spiral out of control and think they're failing! You should weigh yourself weekly at the same time of day, and in the same place, each time, then you'll get an accurate picture. I'd say I weigh myself every few weeks, and each time I go on holiday.'

WHAT YOU'VE LEARNED IN THIS CHAPTER

- That you must learn to live comfortably with food; you have to face it more than once every day.
- Hunger is not a dirty word.
- Don't expect too much too soon.
- Eat mindfully and slowly, and really *taste* your food.
- Food solves nothing except hunger.
- Don't fear failure, learn from it.
- Take responsibility for all your actions.

Chapter 7
Self-Hypnosis 1

In the GMB sessions undertaken at the Elite Clinics, self-hypnosis is a key part of reinforcing the suggestions and images used during therapy. As a reader – if you have the motivation for change – you can achieve similar results and experience that all-important boost to the subconscious through self-hypnosis.

Please note that self-hypnosis should never be practised when driving, operating machinery or carrying out any other activity that requires your full attention.

Self-hypnosis involves relaxing yourself deeply, and thinking yourself through an exercise in which you visualize and reinforce the positive elements of change you're trying to make.

Hypnosis is a state of relaxation – the same kind of feeling you get when you're about to fall asleep at night. Preparing, relaxing; hovering in a twilight zone. Neither awake nor asleep. You are totally aware of outside sounds, but they don't intrude on your state of relaxation. It's a state that's perfectly natural. In fact, you'll have experienced it every day of your life, even if you've never been 'hypnotized'. In hypnosis, your brain is in 'alpha' state – the state in which light sleep and dreams occur.

You're totally in control the whole time – no one's taking control of you. When in this state, your body and mind are very open to suggestions.

You can learn to hypnotize yourself, and provide suggestions to yourself. Your self-induced hypnotic state won't be as deep as is possible when you are hypnotized by someone else, but this is actually necessary because you need to remain aware enough that you can continue to make suggestions to yourself.

Self-hypnosis methods can be used to reduce feelings of anxiety, and to promote feelings of confidence and self-control. *You are going to use self-hypnosis to reinforce a belief in your ability to change your eating patterns for life.*

Choosing Your 'Positive Thoughts'

The self-hypnosis process involves the use of 'Positive Thoughts'. These are statements you use to help develop your subconscious visualization of what you're trying to achieve, and to counteract negative thinking and encourage self-belief. You can choose from our list of Positive Thoughts below, or come up with some of your own. If you choose to do the latter, they should be specifically targeted for each of the three self-hypnosis sessions in the book.

Choose up to three Positive Thoughts that are most relevant and appropriate to you. Then read and revise them, because you need to be able to repeat them silently to yourself at least three times when you're deeply relaxed. They are your messages to your subconscious mind to change your behaviour for life, starting now.

Once you've selected your Positive Thoughts make sure that you feel completely focused on what you're trying to achieve *before* you set about relaxing, so you don't have to refer to notes, or remind yourself what you meant to concentrate on.

It's your subconscious mind you want to target, and that's best addressed when you're deeply relaxed.

If you want to choose a number of Positive Thoughts, you can alternate and select a different set each time you do this session. If you feel you may struggle to remember the words you need to say to yourself, you could consider recording an entire script to play back to yourself when you are ready to go into deep relaxation.

You may decide that you'd prefer to have *all* the Positive Thoughts in your subconscious armoury, and allow yourself as many sessions as necessary to target all of them. If so, keep to the same pattern of choosing a number of Positive Thoughts, relaxing yourself and then repeating them mentally at least three times each.

The Self-Hypnosis Process

Set aside a time each day and find a private, quiet and relaxing area to sit or lie down. Make sure you won't be disturbed, and that all phones are turned off. If you like incense, its scent can help create a specific atmosphere that will become recognizable to your subconscious each time you practise your self-hypnosis. Soft music can be played; use the same track each time. (The use of candles is not advised.)

Lying flat on a bed or couch with arms slightly away from your side is a good starting point. If you choose to place a pillow under your head, it's better to use a fairly flat one so your head and neck aren't strained. Keep your feet and legs uncrossed. If you'd prefer it, you can choose a comfortable chair to sit in. Place your hands flat on your lap or, if your chair has arms, place your arms on them. Keep your spine straight and, again, don't cross your legs or feet.

You now need to 'talk' yourself into a state of deep relaxation.

- You should fix your gaze on a point, so choose something to concentrate on. Then say three or four times, 'I am going to count down from five to one; my eyelids are getting heavy and at one I will close my eyes and be completely relaxed.'

- Now, slowly and silently, count down from five to one, taking a deep breath between each number. When you reach one, close your eyes, and with another, deeper breath, release and relax.

- Now concentrate on every part of your body as a rolling sequence, starting with your feet or your head. Release the tension from each part, and relax your muscles as you go. Repeat silently something like, 'Let go, release, relax'.

- Now picture an evocative set of steps — 10 of them — leading down to somewhere you know you'll be safe and at ease. You can choose — countryside, beach, snowy mountain — it's up to you and your imagination and what makes you feel comfortable.

- Count down from 10 to 1, and at one you should see yourself in that secluded, special place, all alone. Take time to settle down; get used to what's around you — the sounds, the smells, the breeze, tastes… The more you can visualize, the more focused and successful the session will be.

Now imagine yourself standing at a fork in the road of your own life, deciding which path you're going to choose. The left fork is a slippery downhill slope — the low, easy road, the path of least resistance. This is the path you've been going down for many years. The right fork goes slightly uphill – this is the high road. It will take a little bit of effort to follow, because it'll mean making some changes, but it'll also bring many positive benefits.

During the next few minutes you're going to take yourself on a mental journey. First of all, head down the left fork and project your mind forward one year.

Choose your preferred Positive Thoughts from the list below:

1. Remind yourself how bad you feel being out of control – overeating and being overweight.

2. Visualize the rubbish littering the slippery slope – the snack-foods packets and sweet wrappers – and all the emotional pain they are causing you.

3. Catch sight of your reflection in a mirror, looking much older and even bigger.

4. Recognize that if you take this road, you'll be unhappy, your loved ones will be disappointed, your health will be suffering.

5. Feel the weight, not only on your body, but of the disappointment of letting yourself down, of feeling terrible and feeling a failure.

Now bring yourself back to the present day, but remain totally and deeply relaxed – you are going to continue your mental journey. In the next few minutes you're going to head up the right fork and project yourself forward one year.

Take a look at the path ahead of you, and realize it's the road to success – the route to freedom, self-confidence, good health and a longer life.

Choose your preferred Positive Thoughts from the list that follows:

1. This road will lead you to a place where you'll feel better than you have done your whole life: in control and not governed by your food choices.

2. See yourself feeling fantastic – you are fit, healthy, energetic, proud, confident and successful.

3. Spot yourself in a mirror and notice how you look so much younger; you're wearing new clothes; getting admiring glances from your partner and proud looks from your family and friends.

4. Recognize that this is a permanent change – a new way of life.

Now bring yourself back to the present day, but remain totally and deeply relaxed – you are going to complete your mental journey. In the next few minutes you're going to affirm your self-belief and build your confidence in your intention to change.

Choose from these Positive Thoughts:

1. Realize that you're actually still at the fork in the road, but absolutely sure beyond any doubt that you're ready to make the change.

2. The long-term rewards of being slim and healthy far outweigh the instant gratification you used to get from eating the wrong foods for the wrong reasons.

3. From now on, you'll always check to see if you're hungry before you put anything to eat in your mouth.

4. You will never again use boredom or stress as a reason to eat.

5. You will become free to be happier and healthier for the rest of your life – travelling the high road of success.

Having completed all three sets of Positive Thoughts, now count yourself up from one to five, suggesting that you have enjoyed a wonderful relaxation, and on five you will open your eyes, feeling refreshed and energized.

If you decide to do your self-hypnosis before going to sleep, you can suggest that on five you will move into a normal and natural sleep until it's time for you to wake.

As we said earlier, you may decide that you'll relax even more successfully if you don't have to 'remember' your suggestions, or how to talk yourself into deeper relaxation, in which case you could consider buying one of our self-hypnosis CDs (visit www.gmband.com).

Chapter 8

Session 2: Understanding What Your Body Needs

What your body needs, in the long term, is an energy balance. Energy *in* equals energy *out.* Simple. If you consume the same number of calories that your body requires to keep you alive, and carry out whatever activities you do, you'll maintain an even weight.

If you consume fewer calories than your body requires to keep you alive, and sustain whatever physical activity you do, you will lose weight. If you consume more calories than your body needs, you'll gain weight. With barely any exceptions, that's the way it is. Eat more than your body needs, and you'll get fat. Eat less than your body needs, and you'll lose weight.

You've been consuming more than you need – maybe a lot more – for a long time. Now, to drop that weight and learn to maintain an even weight, you need to start consuming fewer calories than you need. Get the long-term energy balance right and your weight, and your sense of wellbeing, will change for the better.

All About Calories

The total energy usage of the human body is determined by four components:

Basal Metabolic Rate (BMR)
This refers to the minimum level of energy needed to sustain vital bodily functions such as breathing, digestion and circulation.[1]

Resting Metabolic Rate (RMR)
A measurement of the number of calories you burn while completely at rest.[2]

Thermic Effect of Food (TEF)
This is the increase in metabolic rate (i.e. the rate at which your body burns calories) that occurs when you've eaten food.[3]

TEA (Thermic Effect of Activity)
This typically accounts for 15 to 30 per cent of the energy you expend in a day, depending on how active you are.[4]

However, none of these — nor any of the other variables such as different muscle mass, hormonal changes, fidgeting, temperature, and so on — makes any fundamental difference to the *overall* picture of how much energy (calories) you burn.

We struggle to understand how anyone can expect to control their weight if they don't know how many calories they're burning. If you feel you'd benefit from knowing what your Resting Metabolic Rate (RMR) is, high-tech tests are relatively inexpensive. At Elite Clinics, for example, we charge €55.

It's possible to get a rough idea of your RMR, though. Multiply your body weight in pounds by 10.5 (or kilograms by 23). For example, someone who weighs 150lb (68kg) has an RMR of around 1,575 calories/day. Scales that feature body composition monitors will also calculate your RMR for you.

Your RMR is the calorific requirement to:

- keep your heart beating and lungs breathing

- keep your internal organs operating properly

- keep your brain functioning

- keep your body warm.

It really helps to have your RMR in mind, because if you're working on allowing yourself around 1,710 calories a day but your body actually only needs 1,575, even allowing for physical activity that's 135 calories each and every day which, over time, you'll be storing as excess weight without ever understanding why.

JUST A SNACK?

A small miscalculation of your calorie intake could add up to a massive weight gain. Let's look at an example. Let's say you eat half a Snickers bar a day on top of what your body needs. Of course, it could also be just one large apple, or a small sandwich, but those 135 extra calories go into your mouth, every day.

How much weight do you imagine you'd have put on at the end of a year? A few pounds? No: a stone; that's

14lbs (6.3kg). 135 calories x 365 days = 49,275 calories you didn't need. And at 3,500 calories a pound (0.45kg), it's not hard to work back. So, if you start when you're 20, by the time you're 40 you could have piled on 280lb (127kg), just by having a snack.

Let's Make it Even Simpler

Your body needs a certain number of calories a day just to exist. Let's say you weigh 200lb (91kg) and your RMR is 2,100 (without even getting out of bed). Providing you're active – walking around the house, playing with the kids, doing the housework, going to work, all the normal activities of daily life – you can eat 2,100 calories a day and lose weight. It's not necessary to restrict yourself to 1,500 or 1,300 calories a day.

The more active you are the quicker you'll lose weight.

But, never forget that, as your weight drops, so does the amount you're able to eat and still lose weight. Say you've lost 7lb (3.2kg) and your RMR is now 2,026. It's not a huge difference, but you have to gradually reduce your portion sizes as you shed the fat.

Scientists have long explored the possible connection between genetics and metabolic rates. There's some fairly old research on mice which suggests there may be a link,[5] but until it's located and proven in humans, and someone develops a way of altering the body's genetic coding to boost what's currently only hereditary low metabolism, we have to work on the knowledge that's presently available.

Getting to Grips with Calories

We started out by suggesting you should learn what your body needs. Maybe now would be a good moment to address your own, probably questionable, understanding of the words 'want' and 'need'. For example, do you *need* that calorie-laden snack, that empty-calorie drink or that fat-soaked meal? Or do you just *want* them?

Get to grips with the difference. Your body needs certain minerals, nutrients, proteins, and so on, but your head and emotions have perhaps been seeking food for other reasons. Don't kid yourself that because you 'need' the crutch of that bar of chocolate that it's a real *physical* need: it's not.

Learn the *real* meaning of want and need and you'll overcome another stumbling block on the route to a healthier body. Make sure you ask yourself the right question — the appropriate question — to peel back the layers of your own deluded thinking. In the end, you need to be asking: 'Does my body physically need this (food, drink) in order to function healthily?' If the answer is no, then it's your choice whether to have it or not.

Do you want to feel how much of a strain you're putting on your body by being overweight? Put your 'excess weight' – in the form of bags of flour or sugar – in a bag or a rucksack. Now pick it up and carry it upstairs with you. Then bring it down again. Now go up again. And down. And so on. How puffed are you?

Now put the bag down and do it again. Do you understand the true meaning of the difference?

With GMB, we don't expect you to count calories day in, day out, for the rest of your life. There's better stuff to do! However, it's useful to have calorie values firmly in the back of your mind as a reference point, so you know, for example, just how disastrous it might be to choose profiteroles over a fruit salad when you order a dessert. And by how much having a double burger and fries could set you back compared to grilled fish and a salad.

So, without getting hung up about it, let's start by looking at how many calories you must have been consuming to get to the weight you are now.

If someone has a sweet tooth and loves chocolate, they probably don't even realize, don't even give it a thought, that a small bar of chocolate – not a family-sized one – can contain 255 calories. It might only amount to a minute of mindless nibbling, but do it every other day, and if it's on top of what your body needs, you'll be looking at an extra stone (6.3kg) on the scales in a year's time.

You could have a nice portion of grilled fish and some vegetables for around the same number of calories as that bar of chocolate, and that's a real meal rather than just a snack. Yet it's amazing that people don't seem to understand this. They look at the calorie content of healthy foods – the things they'd eat as a meal – but not at the calories in cakes, biscuits, etc., because 'they don't count, they're just a snack'.

Therefore, they've no idea how many calories are in just one biscuit, and they deceive themselves. Maybe they'll eat a whole packet over the course of a day – that's as many as 1,000 calories or even more – but convince themselves they haven't eaten much. Instead, they may actually have eaten a whole extra day's worth of calories!

People with an unhealthy attitude to food tend to believe completely illogical concepts. CBT calls these 'sabotaging thoughts', and they're not at all helpful for weight loss. An example of a sabotaging thought would be the belief that whatever you eat while you're standing up – eating on the hoof, perhaps when you're out shopping – doesn't count. It doesn't matter because it's not actually a meal.

The Danger of Hidden Calories

A client returned to the clinic for an 'adjustment session' because she wasn't pleased with her weight loss of less than 1lb (0.45kg) a week. During the course of the session, she told us about the previous evening, when she and her husband had visited a lovely fish restaurant for a low-calorie, healthy meal.

She'd only had a main course – grilled fish and salad, which she knew would be around 275 calories. The couple had ordered a bottle of white wine; she'd drunk about a glass and a half of it, and her husband had the rest. The whole meal was well within her calorie limits – and this scenario wasn't unusual, she said – but still she wasn't losing weight at an acceptable level.

A while later, her husband arrived and he asked how things were going. We said that, based on what his wife had told us about their recent restaurant visit, we were at a loss to understand why she wasn't losing weight very quickly. He then went over what they'd eaten the previous night and told us a different story. We're sure his wife wasn't lying; maybe it was just selective recall!

Before going to the restaurant, he said, they'd visited a bar for a pre-dinner drink. 'Oh, yes,' his wife said, 'I'd forgotten about that.' Then, he said, along with a large glass of wine, his wife had taken quite a few dips into a bowl of peanuts. At the restaurant they were given complimentary tapas while they were looking at the menu. During the meal, his wife put both oil and vinegar on her salad, which she conveniently remembered at that point. And with the bill came complimentary liqueurs.

When we calculated the calorie value of those little 'extras', they added up to almost 900 calories – three times as many as in the low-calorie grilled fish meal.

It's only when someone points these things out that people say, 'Oh, I've been really stupid haven't I?' They might go along merrily saying, 'I haven't eaten anything all day', but actually they had a bar of chocolate, a McDonald's, chips, a milkshake while out shopping… maybe munched some sweets they found in their pocket. But they think those things don't count because they were walking around while they were eating them!

It would take a long while to burn off all those extra calories. You could make up a large fruit salad for less than that one bar of chocolate. You *really* have to question everything you're eating – question your choices.

THE RESTAURANT STING

If you ask 1,000 people if they eat a bread roll before dinner at home, 999 will say no. So why do we go to a restaurant and pay handsomely for an unwanted bread roll? Did we order it? Will it take the edge off our hunger? We actually thank the waitress for giving it to us. Thanks for what? Making us fat? Giving us a carbohydrate addiction? Ensuring that we don't enjoy the meal so much?

Once we start on carbohydrates we can get a craving quite fast; if we have that bread roll before the meal, when we're later offered chips we'll want them – and sticky toffee pudding, the whole works. It's all pre-programmed by us eating the bread roll!

All Calories Are Not Created Equal

A calorie isn't always just a calorie. Many people don't realize that a calorie varies according to the type of food they're eating.[6] Very often, healthier foods contain more fibre, which passes quickly through the body, taking some calories with it (some research suggests that fibre takes fat with it as well). So, a healthy 20-calorie carrot, for example, may 'cost' even fewer calories than that.

In contrast, highly refined, processed foods – those that contain white flour, white sugar and so on – have fewer nutrients and less fibre, so the body absorbs all the calories but gains very little nutritional benefit in the process. So, just by shifting the balance towards healthier foods, you'll not only be consuming fewer calories, but you'll also feel satisfied for much longer.[7] If you eat highly refined foods full of empty calories, you'll not feel satisfied for very long, and as a result, you're more likely to overeat.[8]

When you think about reaching your goal weight – about how much energy and confidence you'll have, the clothes you'll wear and the self-respect you'll gain – how important is it to you? Do you really want it enough?

Face up to the fact that, until now, it hasn't been as appealing or as important to you as the pork pie or the cake.

So, what has to change? What's going to motivate you this time around? You need to find out.

Calories provide us with energy. We obtain a set number of calories from each gram (0.035oz) of carbohydrate, protein, fat and alcohol we consume as this table shows:

1g (0.035oz) portion	Number of calories
Carbohydrate	4
Protein	4
Fat	9
Alcohol	7

Never forget: 1lb (0.45kg) of fat = 3,500 calories; 2.2lbs (1kg) of fat = 7,700 calories.

How Many Calories Are You Consuming?

To give you an idea of the calorie values of some common foods, we compiled the list below. It's a fairly random selection of fruit, vegetables and other foods – you can easily find full calorie-counter lists online if you choose to – but this will give you a general idea of what to avoid, and what to eat more of! (And don't forget to check the labels of shop-bought foods – sugars and fats are often very high on the list of ingredients.

Food	Number of calories
One average-sized apple	60
A small packet of crisps (25g/¾oz)	135
One carrot, boiled	20
Three roast potatoes	210
One portion of roast chicken with gravy	225
Two pieces of toast with butter and marmalade	300

Food	Number of calories
One tomato	25
One Magnum ice cream bar	220
A small carton of plain yoghurt (125g/4½oz)	78
A quarter-pounder burger meal with fries and a small drink	790 (minimum)

For people who are in the process of reducing their weight, alcohol is a multifaceted problem. As we've outlined before, alcohol is believed to increase the appetite, lower resolve and slow the metabolism. Also, it can't be stored by the body, so the body will metabolize it *before* food, leaving any food eaten to be more readily stored as fat.

Did you know that a 250ml (8 fl oz) glass of white wine contains about the same number of calories as four fish fingers?[9] Let's take a look at what you might be quaffing this evening (bear in mind that home measures tend to be significantly larger than standard ones).

Beverage	Number of calories
Double vodka (50ml/1.7 fl oz) and cola	175
Glass of champagne (175ml/6 fl oz)	133
Glass of orange juice (250ml/8 fl oz)	115
Small glass of red wine (125ml/4 fl oz)	85
Large glass of white wine (175ml/6 fl oz)	130
A glass of beer (568ml/1 pint)	180–230
Can of strong lager (500ml/17 fl oz)	225

How to Use Those Calories

Okay, so now you're getting an idea of just how many calories you could be taking in – maybe it's a lot more than your body needs. If you weigh, say, a bit over 19 stone (121kg), simply maintaining your present weight could mean you're eating 3,400 calories a day, or even more – quite a shock?

Of course, you don't want to maintain this weight, you want to decrease it, so you need to be consuming far fewer calories – 500 calories a day fewer than you need for healthy maintenance in order to lose weight at 1lb (0.45kg) a week. So what to do about it?

There are many ways to look at how to deal with the calories you eat, obviously starting with eating fewer than you have been! Two of the most interesting ways are to see how long it takes to burn off a certain number of calories by doing different activities, or how long it would take to 'pay for' a particular food you like! Here are some examples:

Activity	Calories used per hour
Playing knock-about football with friends	560
Messing around on the beach with your children	300
Swimming lengths in a pool	180 (minimum)
Zumba class	500
Digging the garden	340
Cycling (gentle)	300–600
Yoga class	380
Line dancing	311
Intensive aqua-aerobics	295

Activity	Calories used per hour
Driving a vehicle in heavy traffic	80+
Reading; watching TV	70
Grocery shopping; loading and unloading car	165
Moderate walking	225
Housework	146–600 (depending on what it is!)

Remember: everyone burns calories at a different rate according to their weight and metabolism.

We can look at it another way: have you ever wondered how much it would take to 'burn off' something you've just eaten? For example: a glass of red wine = 15 minutes of digging in the garden; a banana = half an hour on a windsurfer; an all-day breakfast = a two-hour walk. Does that put it in some kind of perspective?

If you're looking for a little incentive to move more, you could always buy yourself a pedometer. UK government guidelines suggest that everyone should be walking 10,000 steps a day to maintain good health[10] – and that doesn't take into account any attempt to shift excess weight.

Vitamins, minerals and water add to the nutritional value of the things we consume, but they don't contain any calories. Food and drink that contains few or no nutrients other than the actual foodstuff providing the calories are considered to be a source of 'empty' calories – i.e. they are high in energy (calories), but low in nutritional value as they lack health-promoting 'micro-nutrients' such as vitamins and minerals/antioxidants, and also fibre.

Food and drink containing 'empty' calories includes deep-fried foods such as fries; white bread and white rice; sweets and foods containing added refined sugar; sweetened drinks; fizzy, canned drinks; and alcohol – all wine, beers, spirits, etc.

Choose Superfoods

Try to incorporate some of the so-called 'superfoods' – which contain high levels of antioxidants, fibre, vitamins and minerals – in your diet, along with unprocessed, unrefined foods. You should gradually start to feel health benefits including improved energy levels and immune function, raised mood, and a reduced likelihood of heart disease. Below are just a few of the superfoods:

- Acai berries, goji berries, apples, bananas, apricots, raisins and figs

- Broccoli, watercress and spinach, avocado, Jerusalem artichokes

- Teff grain, hemp, lentils, quinoa, wheatgerm and adzuki beans

- Dark chocolate of 70 per cent or more cocoa solids

- Olive oil

- Salmon

- Natural yoghurt

- Baked beans

- Brazil nuts

- Garlic, ginger and onions

There are others, of course, but if you pick some from this list every day, and discover more for yourself, you'll be on the right lines!

HOW MANY CALORIES ARE YOU REALLY USING?

If you've sat at home all afternoon watching television, you certainly don't need to eat a massive meal in the evening. In fact, you might need to take a good brisk walk to get your metabolism going.

And you've been sitting down reading this book for how long? An hour or so? Any idea how many calories you've used? If you weigh 11st (70kg), it's just 70 calories at the most; at 12st 7lb (79.5kg), it's 80 calories; and if you're 15st (95.5kg) it's 95 calories.

So, not *that* many!

Don't allow yourself to feel that you'll never 'get into' exercise. You only need to make minor changes: park a bit further away from the supermarket; don't take your car right to the door at work; use the stairs instead of the lift as often as you can; walk to the next bus stop. Just don't expect too much of yourself too soon. If you get breathless trying to run for a bus, you're not ready (yet!) to run a marathon. Your fitness will improve over time.

One last thought: you don't need to feel guilty about eating – you need to do it to stay alive! However, even if you're eating healthily, you can still eat too much. Never forget portion size.

All About Portion Control

Now it's time for another reality check. Just knowing how many calories are in pasta, for example, is only half the deal. It's really easy to underestimate exactly how much you're really eating. It's often self-denial and self-delusion – no more, no less. Sitting there and saying, 'I don't eat that much.' Get a grip! You don't put weight on by 'not eating much'. You're obviously overeating and not realizing it, or overeating but refusing to admit to yourself just how bad the problem is.

He that eats until he is sick must fast until he is well.
HEBREW PROVERB

In the early days of GMB research, we ran a test on friends to establish when people were satisfied with a meal. Three couples joined us for dinner at our home and filled in a little questionnaire the following day. Each couple was served an identical fresh pasta meal; the only difference was the portion size. The plates varied in size from 'small' to large, restaurant-sized pasta dishes. The portion sizes were calculated to fill each plate/dish.

On night number one, we served a portion of the size we would normally have for dinner after work at home: around 80g (3oz) of (dried, uncooked) pasta per head. The plates were cleared; everyone enjoyed the food. On the second night, Marion produced portions for the next couple, which were weighed at 160g (5½ oz); once again the plates were cleared and the food enjoyed. On the final night, Marion served portions in pasta dishes loaned by our favourite Italian restaurant. We also used the restaurant's portion sizes, which were an amazing 260g (9oz). Guess what? The plates were cleared, the food enjoyed.

One of the questions we asked the couples was, 'Did you go home feeling sufficiently full?' All three couples said yes, even though the last one's portion size was nearly three times that of the first. We wondered, *do we eat until we are full? Until we are tired? Or maybe until the plate is empty, regardless?*

When you're calculating the calorie value of what you've eaten, you might think you've had a spoonful of this, a little bit of that, but if you actually *measured* the portions, you'd probably find that you'd eaten about two or three times more than you thought you had.

How about a bowl of cereal – have you ever calculated the calorie value of your portion? You might think it's 200 calories, including the milk, but we know from clients that, in reality, you probably have double the recommended serving size. So, before you're even out the door in the morning, you've consumed twice as many calories as you thought you had. If you're doing that every day, with every meal, all those guesstimates and miscalculations have added up, and they're showing on the scales right now.

People have different opinions on the value of eating breakfast, but overnight is usually the longest period you'll go without eating. Okay, so you're not doing much – just resting – but if you wake up not feeling hungry, you're probably eating too much.

THE MOST IMPORTANT MEAL OF THE DAY?

There are some who believe we should 'breakfast like a king, lunch like a prince, dine like a pauper'. Some nutritionists might agree with this principle, but on the basis of how and when energy and nutrients are needed and used during a 24-hour period!

Clinical trials have proven that a high-protein breakfast,[11] such as eggs, keeps hunger pangs away for much longer than a carbohydrate-based breakfast such as toast or cereal. Porridge is officially the most satisfying cereal: it has a higher protein content than any other grain and is also a good source of soluble fibre.

It's so easy to fall down when it comes to portion sizes. Dressings are another pitfall. You might say that you just had a salad for lunch. But what did you put on it? Just a bit of oil and vinegar? But if you calculate exactly how much oil you used, you'd probably be quite surprised – there could be more calories in the dressing than in the salad itself. It's about being aware. We need to eat *some* fat – and olive oil is good for us – but, just because something is healthy, it doesn't mean we should consume unlimited quantities of it.

You can save yourself a lot of calories by easing off the oil in your dressing and adding balsamic vinegar – 1 tablespoon (15ml) of vinegar contains just 16 calories. How much butter do you put on your bread or toast? If you love butter, fair enough, but make sure you have it for the flavour, not the quantity. It all adds up, and it shows on the scales.

Even healthy foods like nuts and seeds are very high in calories, so it's easy to get carried away. A small, 115g (4oz) bag of nuts contains up to 800 calories. But you wouldn't count that as a meal, would you? You'd probably think of it as a snack! So, again, it's all about being aware of quantities. Two tablespoons (30g) of nuts amounts to a standard portion of protein; that's a small handful, around 150 calories – not a whole bag!

Do you like ice cream? A scoop of ice cream contains about 150 calories, but you may eat twice or three times that amount – that's quite a chunk of your daily energy requirement in one go. And eating it with a spoon straight out of the container (don't say you haven't done this!) means you have no idea how much you're having. Take the container out of the freezer, measure it into a dish, put the rest back, and when that portion's gone, it's gone!

Doesn't dried pasta look small? So you put more in, and then, when it's cooked, the temptation is to eat it all up rather than 'waste' it. Instead, it's better not to cook too much in the first place! A portion of cooked pasta should be about the size of a woman's fist. That uncooked, 80g (3oz) serving – very much depending on the shape of the pasta – will be about as much as a woman can hold in the palm of her hand. It's not uncommon for people to eat three times that amount, and this also happens in Italian restaurants. You have a massive pile of pasta on your plate, and you just don't need that much. Then, of course, there's the high-calorie sauce.

DON'T BE THE BIN!

I must eat that last piece of cake or pizza or it will only go to waste. It's something we've all said or thought many times. But have we *really* thought it through? If you don't eat it, it'll go in the bin – go to landfill. And if you do eat it? Well, whether your body needs it or not, the majority of it will pass through your digestive system down the toilet via the sewerage system and possibly to landfill. Is that what the word 'waste' means?

Why don't you just buy less food in the first place? Then you won't have those leftovers facing you in the fridge!

Don't treat your body like a bin. You deserve better.

Getting to Grips with Portion Sizes

The good thing about portion control is, once you've got your head around it, you can eat *whatever* you want. For the rest of your life. It is *way better* than dieting and you don't need to have 'forbidden' foods.

Do you understand? Read that again. In fact we'll say it again: 'You don't need to have forbidden foods. Eat whatever foods you want to eat.' The point being, if you understand portion control, you can eat whatever you choose. If you're aware of what's high in calories and you particularly want to eat it, as long as you have a *small* portion of it, in the end it's not going to do any damage.

Then, looking at the bigger picture, if you're eating sensibly for most of the time, you can 'afford' to eat a *bit* more of the calorie-laden foods on one day a week, or two days a fortnight. *Don't do it more often than that, though!*

It's all about achieving a balance: a reasonable combination of healthy foods with a few less healthy ones when you occasionally feel you want them!

You know that if you eat out and have a two-course meal with wine that you're likely to consume about 20 per cent more than in an average meal you have at home, so you can 'budget' for that over the course of the week. For example, you know that Sunday is going to be a blowout, so what you do is go easy on the Saturday, and on the Monday afterwards – a couple of days either side compensates and balances things out.

Eating out doesn't have to be a disaster, but it does require you to see the overall picture. This is what normal-weight people do naturally anyway.

*See every encounter with food as a game,
a contest; there will always be a winner or
a loser, so don't be the victim all your life.*

We try to instil in people the understanding that there's absolutely nothing wrong with enjoying food and eating. You *can* love food and follow the GMB system. We do. Marion – yes, slim, size 8 Marion – loves food, loves cooking and the wonderful stimulus of eating and dining with friends.

You don't need to deprive yourself of anything. If you want something, have it, *but only eat it if you're hungry.* It's when you eat food when you're *not* hungry that the problems start. People often feel guilty about what they've eaten because they know they weren't actually hungry in the first place. When you're eating for the right reason, though, there's no need to feel guilty about it. As long as you're eating a healthy, balanced diet overall, you can have all the extra things too, in moderation. It's all about moderation and portion control.

*'I found the whole GMB experience enlightening,
and I was losing weight steadily, whereas before it
was a huge struggle. I was more conscious of what
I was eating, and how. I noticed when I was full, and
was able to leave food when I had that feeling.'*
GMB client **J.S.**

How to Measure a Portion

If you don't have measuring spoons and measuring cups and scales, you really don't need to go out and buy a whole new set of kitchen equipment to gauge the portion sizes you should be eating. Read on and we'll show you an easier way.

There are variations in the standard metric and imperial methods used for measuring liquid, dry or solid ingredients, so the figures given here are approximate, but sufficiently accurate to get you on your way with understanding quantities.

If you're going to get to grips with how much food to put on your plate, or put in the pan in the first place, should you use scales? You can if you want to – some people prefer to be painstakingly accurate in order to teach themselves. However, others find that visual aids which allow them to imagine the size or shape of something are helpful. To this end, we've compiled a list of objects to help you *picture* the quantities you prepare for yourself.

Think of the following:

- A domino

- A dice

- A pack of playing cards/a woman's palm

- A cheque book

- A golf ball

- A tennis ball/a child's fist

- A walnut

- A hazelnut in its shell

- A woman's fist

- The tip of a thumb

Sometimes it's easier to gauge an amount if you can visualize another object that's the equivalent size and dimensions. Here are the ones we use:

1 teaspoon (5g/5ml) = a dice, a domino, a hazelnut in its shell, or the tip of a thumb
1 tablespoon (15g/15ml) = a walnut, three thumb tips

One teaspoon (5g) of butter spread on your toast contains 35 calories; one tablespoon (15g) contains 105 calories. With the teaspoon, the toast will have butter thinly spread all over it, without any gaps; with the tablespoon the butter will not be spread, but thickly pasted on the bread.

One teaspoon (5g) of mayonnaise contains about 30 calories, whereas 1 tablespoon (15g) has 90, so being over-generous with the dressing can end up doubling the number of calories in a healthy, low-calorie salad!

Just one extra tablespoon (15ml) of oil each day amounts to a weight gain of a stone (6.3kg) over the course of a year!

38g/60ml/¼ cup = a golf ball
Nuts: 38g (¼ cup) of walnuts contains 155 calories

75g/120ml/½ cup = a tennis ball or a child's fist
Ice cream: 120ml (½ cup) of ice cream contains 150 calories, so twice that amount, 240ml (1 cup), of ice cream adds a massive 300 calories onto your daily intake!

150g/240ml/1 cup = a woman's fist
Pasta: 150g (1 cup) of cooked pasta contains around 250–300 calories.
About 80g (3oz) of dried pasta = 150g (1 cup) when cooked (beware: the volume of pasta varies a lot depending on its shape).

Proteins (meat and fish)

Ideally, you should aim to eat two to three portions of protein per day. These can be meat and/or fish, or alternative sources such as pulses (peas, beans, lentils). Other protein-rich foods include nuts, seeds and eggs.

A standard portion of meat is 80g (3oz) = a pack of playing cards/a woman's palm

80g (3oz) of chicken breast, roasted without the skin = 140 calories
80g (3oz) of lean fillet steak = 170 calories

A standard portion of fish is 115–140g (4–5oz) = a cheque book

140g (5oz) of cod, hake or snapper baked or steamed = 130 calories
80g (2¾ oz) can of tuna = 103 calories

Other proteins

1 egg = 90 calories
75g (2½ oz) cooked lentils = 120 calories
100g (3½ oz) cooked chickpeas = 164 calories

Dairy products

Sample adult portion sizes are: 200ml (7 fl oz) of milk; 150ml (5 fl oz) of yoghurt; 40g (1½ oz) hard cheese; 90g (3¼ oz) cottage cheese. The average recommended daily consumption of dairy products is three portions.
28g (1oz) hard cheese = 110 calories
50g (1¾ oz) cottage cheese = 49 calories
284ml (½ pint) whole milk = 70 calories; semi-skimmed = 50 calories

Carbohydrates

Carbs should make up 45–65 per cent of your total daily intake; complex carbs, such as fresh fruit and vegetables, are better for you than refined carbs: sugar, white flour, white rice.

150g (1 cup) of ready-to-eat cereal, e.g. cornflakes = 101 calories

Baked potato – one large (335g/12oz) = 278 calories

Bread – one slice from a medium brown loaf = 82 calories; white = 100 calories

Rice – white. A 75g (2½ oz) portion of dry rice swells during cooking to approximately one cup of cooked rice, which serves two people and contains 380 calories.

Pasta – white. A 160g (5¾ oz) portion of dry pasta is enough to serve two people when cooked, and contains 482 calories.

Fresh fruit and vegetables

The average recommended daily consumption of fruit and vegetables is five portions.

An average adult portion is 80g (3oz) = a pack of playing cards/a woman's palm

1 banana = 112 calories

1 apple = 62 calories

1 peach/nectarine = 35 calories

2 satsumas = 58 calories

Honeydew melon, one 125g (4½ oz) slice = 36 calories

15 grapes = 45 calories

Broccoli – 100g (3½ oz) cooked = 32 calories

Carrots – 100g (3½ oz) cooked = 32 calories

Sweet corn – 100g (3½ oz) cooked = 24 calories

Cabbage – 100g (3½ oz) cooked = 24 calories

Green beans – 100g (3½ oz) cooked = 25 calories

Celery – 1 stalk = 6 calories

Cucumber – 1 whole medium = 45 calories

Pyramid, Pie Chart or Plateful?

Food is fuel. It's not an emotional crutch, nor something to fill a boring life. It's just a fuel. Ideally, as you do for your car, you'll choose the best fuel for the job – full of the right nutrients to run your body healthily and efficiently (though a *little* of what you fancy can do you good!). This fuel, a bit like unleaded petrol or diesel, is full of all sorts of ingredients. Unlike petrol or diesel, though, it's not really possible to buy a perfectly nutritious diet in one go off a forecourt, so it helps if you have an idea of the various elements you should be including, and in what proportions.

A pyramid, or a pie chart, is often used to indicate which foods you should eat more of, and those you should consume less of. Maybe, though, it's more realistic to see this as a plate full of food – in the way that you look down at your own plate in front of you at mealtimes. You can think of that plate as your day's requirements – a health-giving 'tankful'!

In descending order of quantity, your plate should contain: **Mostly** Fruit and vegetables; **Less** Bread, cereals and potatoes; **Less again** Milk and dairy products; **Even less** Meat and fish; **The smallest amount** Foods containing saturated fats and refined sugars.

A FISTFUL OF FOOD

While you've got the image of a plate in mind, you might like to consider this visual reminder of portion sizes. Your stomach capacity is about one fistful of food, once it's been chewed. To produce that, a typical sensible portion size is two fists. So if you eat more than two fists of food at any meal you're overeating!

Beige Food versus Rainbow Food

We like to call 'junk' food – the low-nutrient, easy-to-eat, high-fat, high-sugar, quick-fix food loved by so many overweight people – 'beige food'. Avoid beige food and you'll not only be helping the weight-loss process, but upping your vitamin and mineral intake too. Beige food consists mainly of 'empty calories'. Examples include crisps, chips, cakes, biscuits, white bread, white rice and white pasta.

By contrast, foods that are healthy and unprocessed will often also be quite colourful – when you think about it, you don't see many beige-coloured fruit or vegetables, do you? In general, the more vivid the colour of a food, the more nutritious it is.

How about seeing fruit and vegetables as a rainbow of nutrition, and do your best to include a good mix of colours at every meal?[12] Here's a very brief overview of some of the health benefits of rainbow foods:

Red: tomatoes, strawberries, raspberries, red onion, pomegranates, etc. These improve memory function, urinary tract health, and heart health.

Orange: carrots, pumpkins, mangoes, oranges, etc. Good for the eyes and skin, these foods also protect against infection and boost the immune system.

Yellow: bananas, papayas, yellow peppers, pineapples, sweet corn. Good for teeth and gums, they prevent inflammation, aid circulation, and help cuts to heal.

Green: broccoli, limes, apples, lettuce, kiwi fruit. These are good for eyesight, the bones, the teeth, and circulation.

Blue/purple: grapes, plums, aubergines, red cabbage, red lettuce. Good for circulation, the heart, memory function, and urinary tract health.

White: ginger, cauliflower, mushrooms, parsnips. Good for lowering cholesterol levels, joint health, and the prevention of cancer and heart disease.

> 'GMB was all very easy – almost unbelievably. You just have to do it. I looked at food as calories, and asked myself if they were worth adding to my daily intake.'
> **GMB CLIENT ARTHUR**

All About Water

Water is a vital ingredient in a healthy diet. It plays a sometimes confusing part in weight loss, though, not least because, as we said earlier, it's easy to mistake the body's signals for needing water as a sign of hunger. This confusion intensifies with increasing age.[13] Signs that the body is dehydrated include dizziness, headache, fatigue, fuzzy short-term memory and the sensation of extreme hunger.[14] So we often end up reaching for food when all we really needed was a drink – the hunger was just thirst in disguise!

Water is actually more important to us than food; we can survive for a month or so without food, but only a few days without water.

The human body is over 55 per cent water, and on a daily basis we can lose up to 4 litres (7 pints) through urine, sweat and exhaled breath. If you add in exercise, or living in a hot climate, water loss increases dramatically.[15]

Hunger is just thirst in disguise!

It's vital to drink water for your body to function properly. It will make you feel fitter and more energetic, as well as reducing the likelihood of 'dehydration' headaches. Dehydration can cause a dip in your metabolic rate of up to 3 per cent,[16] so not only is drinking fresh (calorie-free!) water good for your body, it's also a great way of ensuring it uses up those calories at the optimum rate.

Water is an essential part of our digestive system, and performs the following functions: [17]

- Dissolves and transports waste products from the cells.

- Makes up more than half our blood, most of our brain and muscle; even 20 per cent of bone is water.

- Transports nutrients and waste products in the blood and lymphatic systems.

- Is a component of sweat, helping the body maintain a constant temperature.

- Protects, cushions and lubricates organs, joints and the colon.

How much water do you need to drink? Well, it depends on your body weight. Generally, for roughly every 2lbs (1kg) of body weight, you need 0.03 litres (1oz) of water. So, if you weigh 10st 3lb (65kg), you should drink 2.15 litres (3¾ pints) of water a day.[18] Weigh rather more than that? At 14st 2lb (90kg), you'll need around 3 litres (5¼ pints).

WATER AND LOW-CARB DIETS

The reason you lose weight quickly in the first stages of a low-carbohydrate diet is because the body stores sugar (glycogen) along with three times its weight in water.[19] If you use up a lot of the glycogen stores – which is quite likely if your food intake is cut dramatically – the water is shed along with the glycogen. However, if you return to your old eating habits after the diet, the glycogen is likely to come back, along with its water!

If you're losing weight sensibly, at 1–2lb (450–900g) a week, as with GMB, this is unlikely to happen.

We tend to think that we're getting our water intake by drinking any fluid that contains water, such as tea, coffee, alcohol, and other manufactured beverages. However, while it's true that these beverages *do* contain water, what can happen is that their other ingredients can sometimes *deprive* the body of more water than has been consumed, leaving you even more dehydrated. The most effective way to replenish your water level is by drinking fresh water. Most fresh fruit and vegetables are made up of between 70 and 95 per cent water, so eating plenty of these will help up your daily intake.

If you keep a bottle of water with you, you can take regular sips throughout the day. If you wait until your mouth is dry, and you feel thirsty, it means you're already dehydrated, and this is the final signal that the body urgently needs water. A good sign that you are getting enough water is when your urine has either very little or no colour to it, and is odourless. If it's dark yellow and strong smelling, you should drink more water.

It makes it a lot easier for you, psychologically, to meet your daily water intake if you use a small bottle. It's handy to keep with you at all times, and is much more portable than a large bottle. Every small step adds up to a big result in the end!

All About Exercise

You'll hear it said that today's obese generation(s) could be forgiven for eating too much because they haven't been taught to recognize that they do so much less exercise than their parents or grandparents.[20] Not so many years ago, we had to get up from the sofa and walk over to the TV to select a different channel. Now we have remote controls that can do just about everything except make the tea or coffee.

Our mothers had to use push-along carpet sweepers, but today we not only have high-powered vacuum cleaners, but some of us have even done away with the bag, as it uses so much energy, time and effort to go out and buy and then install a replacement!

In the same way, no one *carries* heavy suitcases any more; they now often come with two wheels – sometimes four. Cars have power steering and electric windows; some even have electric wing mirrors and electric systems for moving the seat! All of this, combined with longer working hours, a greater use of household gadgets, and a reliance on cars and public transport, may be a factor in the (literally) ballooning nature of our obese population.

Many of our clients say that their eating habits have become ingrained because of what they were taught or shown as a child. We try to get them to see that they're using 'selective memory': they no longer believe in Santa Claus, the Easter Bunny, or the Tooth Fairy, but they do tend to stick with their nice 'supper before bedtime', just like they did with their mum and dad. Convenient really!

However, something has to happen, and happen now. If you're one of those prepared to take responsibility for your size, and do something about it, read on.

By now, you've established:

- more or less, how many calories you need to keep yourself alive.

- how many calories you may be eating compared with how many you should be eating.

- how many calories are in various foods, so you can begin to change your eating habits.

- the portion sizes that will help you cut down that intake.

- that you mustn't forget to drink water.

Okay, Let's Get Moving

Few people love it, many of us hate it, but we've all got to do more of it. Let's take a look now at how exercise can play a part in your GMB journey.

If you've not really been doing any exercise at all, or you used to and have now stopped, there's no point in suddenly hoping to do loads of stuff you really don't like. You won't magically enjoy going to the gym if you detest the idea of it in the first place.

If you love the gym, that's brilliant. But if you find that having all those Lycra-clad folk around you makes you depressed, you have plenty of alternatives. You could walk around the block – that burns calories. Throw sticks for your dog in the park – it'll make both of you happy *and* burn calories. You could go to a salsa class with your friends and have a good giggle (and burn calories).

Just find something you like that keeps you moving and gets your heart rate up! Oh, and if you try something and then decide it's not for you after all, by all means give it up, but don't give up on exercise. Find something else to do. So kickboxing wasn't for you? Try the tango!

In order to shed one pound (0.45kg) a week, you need to

eat 500 calories a day *less* than your body needs for whatever activity level you have. You can do this by simply eating less, but it'll help if you include some exercise in your daily routine – it's good for your heart, lungs, circulation, skin, etc., and exercise increases your metabolism temporarily, which means that, during the exercise and for up to 24 hours afterwards, you'll be burning calories faster (only very slightly though, maybe a couple of dozen calories a time).

Exercising regularly doesn't happen without a bit of effort. You'll know from reading this far that positive thinking achieves so much more than negativity. This applies to exercise, too. If you start today, you may not have Halle Berry's flat abs, or Michelle Obama's toned arms, by next week, but you'll be a step closer, and what we do today affects how we feel tomorrow. Sooner rather than later those wobbly bits will be a bit less wobbly!

The trick is to take it slowly. Bit by bit you'll form a healthy exercise habit to add to the healthy eating habits you're developing. It'll be your choice, and your choice alone, to take control of the problem that's made you uncomfortable and unhappy for so long.

> **Keep this in mind next time you're feeling tempted to reach for an unhealthy 'snack': you would have to spend 48 minutes doing sit-ups to work off the calories contained in one McDonald's Big Mac meal![21]**

> **And it takes more than an hour of housework to burn the calories in just half a Snickers 2 To Go bar!**

Everyone burns calories at different rates during exercise, as they do when at rest. The heavier you are, the more calories you'll use, so, actually, the more excess weight you have to shift, the harder you have to work to use up calories! It takes quite some time to 'burn' calories in some everyday activities, so by far the best way to achieve long-term weight loss is to follow our suggested route of eating smaller, sensible quantities of food, eating only when you're hungry, and generally increasing your level of exercise.

Let's look at it another way. Try to incorporate one or more of the following activities into your day; each will use 100 calories:

- A brisk walk.

- 30 minutes playing with your children, or maybe doing some housework.

- A bit of light gardening.

- Some aerobics with your as-yet-unused aerobics DVD.

- Cleaning out the garage.

Strategies for Moving More

We've been talking about all the elements to consider if you're going to change your relationship with food. Your attitude, your choices, your ability to question each and every thing you are about to eat, should now start to change overnight. They may not change *enough* immediately – it can take time to unlearn deeply ingrained habits – but you are likely to see a change very quickly.

Once you've left food on your plate once, it'll be increasingly easy to do again. Pride at doing that breeds confidence, which creates a virtuous circle. At mealtimes, learning to eat your favourite foods first rather than last saves piling through a plateful of things you are not overly keen on. Simple lessons, easily learned – once you know how!

So, you should leave a restaurant having enjoyed your meal because you've eaten your favourite food, and you haven't forced anything into your mouth that you weren't going to enjoy anyway: you've stopped at a comfortable level rather than eating the whole lot. It's just a completely different way of looking at things.

Another interesting approach to weight loss is to 'pay for your food in advance'. Basically, this means you can eat whatever you want, as long as you choose some form of exercise to do *first*, in order to burn off the number of calories contained in it. Once you've done the exercise, you can either allow yourself to have that tempting cheeseburger, chocolate bar, cake, whatever, knowing that it won't actually cause you to put on weight. Of course, you can choose *not* to eat it, and as a result you'll be really pleased with your efforts, knowing that you've worked off those calories that'll help you achieve your desired outcome of being slimmer.

There's yet another way of looking at how to use exercise to help lose excess weight. Say you've just had a 'snack attack' and devoured a whole chocolate bar. Some 350 calories, all in one go. You could go for a brisk walk for an hour and twenty minutes – that'd get rid of it. *Or* you could go for that walk for 30 minutes, and that would make it seem as if you'd only eaten a bit more than half the chocolate. Every little helps!

In case there's still doubt in your mind that you've got to cut down on those high-fat, high-calorie junk and comfort foods, think about what you'd have to do to 'get rid of' some of your favourites:

- 1 teaspoon (5g) sugar = scrubbing the floor for two minutes
- 1 digestive biscuit = walking up the stairs for eight minutes
- 28g (1oz) crisps = jogging for 12 minutes
- A 85g (3oz) bar of milk chocolate = nearly two hours of housework!

Many people think that gradual weight gain is a fact of life. Well, although it's often seen as some kind of joke, it's true that metabolism decreases by about 2 per cent per decade after the age of 30 – mainly due to loss of muscle mass as our bodies age.[22] So, finding ways to maintain your muscle mass can help keep your metabolism working faster.

Never forget that the heavier you are, the more calories you burn and, conversely, as you shift the excess weight, the fewer calories you burn, so you need to do more exercise to achieve the same result.

One pound (0.45kg) of lean muscle burns very slightly more calories than the equivalent in fat, so a muscular person is more likely to have a higher Resting Metabolic Rate (RMR). The assertion that 'muscle weighs more than fat' is obviously illogical. The reason people have this idea is because muscle is about 18 per cent more dense than fat, so it takes up less space.[23] A person with a higher percentage of muscle will not only have a faster metabolism than one carrying a lot of body fat, they will also look more streamlined.

Let's look at the implications for a snacker of just sitting and watching TV – something that we all do rather too much of these days. Let's say they watch one soap opera a week and during the show they eat a packet of crisps – that's 5lb (2.26kg) a year excess weight. A glass of wine to wash the crisps down? That's another 2lb (0.9kg) a year.

So that one soap a week adds up to half a stone (over 3kg) by the end of the year. On top of this, researchers have found that diners who are distracted by a TV feel hungry sooner than those who eat a meal at a table and concentrate on enjoying the taste of the food.[24]

SUPERHUMANS

When in motion, the human body uses energy very efficiently. A person running a marathon (26 miles/42km) only burns about 2,600 calories – about 100 calories per mile.[25] A typical car achieves between 15 and 50 miles (24–80km) to the gallon; and a gallon of petrol (about half a litre) contains about 31,000 calories. This means that if a human could drink petrol to take in calories instead of eating food, they could run a marathon on only one-twelfth of a gallon of petrol.[26]

In other words, a human being gets more than 300 miles (482km) to the gallon!

Take a Jar of Fat

If you want to give yourself a real shock, try this – a visual incentive for weight loss if ever there was one! Find yourself two glass jars: one small, one larger, with screw-top lids, and then buy a couple of packets of lard. Soften (but don't melt) the lard and then put about half an ounce (15g) in the small jar and 1lb (0.45kg) in the larger jar, and seal the lids. You've just made yourself a reminder of what 1lb (0.45kg) of fat looks like – that's 3,500 calories. The little jar – with its tiny quantity – contains 100 calories.

Carry the smaller jar with you in your handbag or coat pocket. Each time you grab a couple of handfuls of crisps, that's over 100 calories gone just like that. And if those 100 calories are on top of what your body needs, they'll become what you have in that small jar – fat. It'll be quite a wake-up call!

Say you're 1lb (0.45kg) lighter at the end of a week, instead of being disappointed, look at the 1lb jar and you'll know how much fat you've shed. Excess weight that you're no longer carrying around with you. Maybe if you put the jar on top of the fridge it would remind you every time you went for something to eat!

So, with that jar of fat fresh in your mind, stop and imagine two arteries – one clear, belonging to a healthy person, the other clogged up with fatty deposits. (If you've ever seen a furred-up pipe, you'll have some idea what a clogged artery looks like – it's not a pretty sight.) What should be a clear route for your blood to course around your body, carrying oxygen one way and carbon dioxide the other, becomes narrower and narrower as the fat deposits build up, making the heart work unnecessarily hard.

What comes next? Well, a heart attack is a distinct possibility; death is another. And medical opinion is divided on the chances of actually reversing the damage. Think again about that gloopy, marbled fat, creating harder and harder work for your poor heart. Not nice, and totally avoidable. So why do you do it?

'Marion's questions made me face up to the fact that my behaviour had become self-destructive, and that I was actually choosing to make myself fat. That night, I wrote

in my diary, "This stops here." And it did. From that moment on, I changed the way I thought about food. The strong, no-bullshit approach from Martin gave me practical advice for making permanent change.'

GMB CLIENT JACQUIE

WHAT YOU'VE LEARNED IN THIS CHAPTER
. . . .

- It's useful to know your Resting Metabolic Rate (RMR), so you can estimate how much you should be eating.

- Eat more than your body needs = get fat. Eat less than your body needs = shift weight.

- To think of alcohol as 'empty' calories.

- Cooking too much food is waste on your waist.

- To go easy on dressings and sauces.

- Good portion control = no forbidden foods.

- How to visualize portion sizes.

- How to make water your friend.

- Hunger is just thirst in disguise.

- Calorie counting is unnecessary and boring, but an understanding of food values is vital.

- You can 'pay for your food' in advance.

- Eat less and move more!

- To picture that jar of fat when you find yourself reaching for junk food.

Chapter 9
Self-Hypnosis 2

In Self-Hypnosis 1 we explained how, with the motivation for change, you can provide yourself with a boost to the subconscious by relaxing deeply. If you want to remind yourself of the process, you will find it on page 119.

Please note that self-hypnosis should never be practised when driving, operating machinery or carrying out any other activity that requires your full attention.

For this session, choose up to three Positive Thoughts from the list below that are relevant and appropriate, and read and revise them. You need to be able to repeat them silently to yourself at least three times. They are your messages to your subconscious to change your behaviour for life, starting now.

If there are more than three appropriate Positive Thoughts, you can alternate and choose a different set each time you do this session.

Read your 'Positive Thoughts' and make sure you feel completely focused on what you are trying to achieve before you set about relaxing, so you don't have to open your eyes to refer to notes, or remind yourself what you meant to concentrate on.

It's the subconscious mind you want to target, and that is best addressed when you are deeply relaxed.

- You should fix your gaze on a point, so choose something to concentrate on. Then say three or four times, 'I am going to count down from five to one; my eyelids are getting heavy and at one I will close my eyes and be completely relaxed.'

- Now, slowly and silently, count down from five to one, taking a deep breath between each number. When you reach one, close your eyes, and with another, deeper breath, release and relax.

- Now concentrate on every part of your body as a rolling sequence, starting with your feet or your head. Release the tension from each part, and relax your muscles as you go. Repeat silently something like, 'Let go, release, relax'.

- Now picture an evocative set of steps – 10 of them – leading down to somewhere you know you'll be safe and at ease. You can choose – countryside, beach, a snowy mountain – it's up to you and your imagination and what makes you feel comfortable.

- Count down from 10 to 1, and at one you should see yourself in that secluded, special place, all alone. Take time to settle down; get used to what's around you – the sounds, the smells, the wind, tastes… The more you can visualize, the more focused and successful the session will be.

As you relax, you are now confident that you are at last on the journey to conquering your bad relationship with food. Stop and think for a moment how good you feel that your figure no longer needs to be a constant worry. Feel good that you have taken the first step.

During the next few minutes, you're going to take yourself on a mental journey to see just how much you've changed and will continue to change.

Picture yourself sitting down to eat a healthy, balanced meal. Thinking through the process of producing smaller meals, and serving them on smaller plates. Focusing your attention on your food; eating slowly and mindfully; taking smaller mouthfuls; swallowing and completely emptying your mouth before you take another forkful. Occasionally putting your fork down, and checking if you're really hungry before eating any more.

Then picture yourself at your target weight, focusing your attention on the positive feelings that go with being slim. If you find yourself reaching for food when you're not hungry, your subconscious will distract you into doing something else.

Remind yourself by repeating your Positive Thoughts. For this session, choose at least three suggestions from this list:

1. My stomach is much smaller and I feel completely satisfied eating less food.

2. I'm choosing to eat healthily much more often now.

3. I eat slowly and mindfully and chew each mouthful thoroughly.

4. I'm choosing to drink plenty of pure, fresh water every day.

5. I'm choosing to drink less alcohol.

6. I only eat in response to physical hunger now, and not for any other reason.

7. I stop eating as soon as I feel lightly satisfied.

8. I have no need or desire to eat until I feel stuffed full, or my plate is empty.

9. I'm in control of what I eat and how I eat.

10. I eat in order to live and food has no control over me.

11. I feel calm and relaxed about food and eating.

12. I love and respect my body and treat it with the love and respect it deserves.

13. My energy levels are increasing, and I want to be more active.

14. I feel positive, and confident that I can achieve and maintain my ideal weight.

Now count yourself up from one to five, suggesting that you have enjoyed a wonderful relaxation, and on five you will open your eyes, feeling refreshed and energized.

If you decide to do your self-hypnosis before going to sleep, you can suggest that on five you will move into a normal and natural sleep until it's time for you to wake.

Chapter 10

Session 3: Weight Loss in Five Words

In order to give yourself the best possible start on your GMB weight-loss journey, now is the time to remember five key words. Write them down if it helps, but make sure you remember them one way or another.

- **Hunger**

  Do you know what it really means to *you*? Do you go long enough without eating to experience it? Do you know the symptoms of true hunger? You should eat when and only because you are hungry.

- **Fullness**

  Can you stop eating *before* you are full? Have you learned to eat more slowly, to give your brain time to catch up with your body's signals? Have you understood the concept of stopping eating when you are 80 per cent full and no more?

- **Want** and **Need**

  Do you *want* that food or drink (whatever it may be!) or do you actually *need* it, for your body and health, because you are hungry?

- **Motivation**

  Have you identified *why* you want to take steps to shed your excess weight? Until you've fully understood your own reasons, it's likely to be an uphill battle. Motivation is key.

When you were completing the questionnaire in Chapter 6 we asked you to be honest in your answers; GMB requires you to be brutally honest with yourself, even if it feels uncomfortable. The problems around your unhealthy relationship with food have probably existed for a long time and require addressing in order for you to proceed. You'll be surprised at what you can learn about yourself and your life from your eating habits.

Hopefully, by just slowly and quietly asking yourself the questions, and thinking about your possible answers, you may already be starting to think differently about what and why you are eating.

At the clinic we're constantly monitoring clients' weight-loss results, and asking ourselves and each other the same question: 'Why did *that* person just breeze through the treatment, and consistently lose weight week on week, while another client of the same age and the same level of obesity continues to struggle, or even fail?'

The answer in many cases comes back to one word: motivation. It's such a simple word and one that initially even *we* failed to devote sufficient time to. When we ask a client what their main reasons are for wanting to lose weight, what we are really asking is, 'What would motivate you to change?' They come up with a wide range of answers.

Ask Yourself the Right Questions

We have learned to always question the first reason clients give us for wanting to lose weight. Often it's not the *real* reason – not to begin with, anyway. If someone says they want to do it for their health, we say, 'Okay, if you could take a tablet and then be healthy and live a full and active life, would you still want to lose weight?' They'll say, 'Well, actually yes, because I want to feel more attractive for my partner,' or 'I want to be able to wear more fashionable clothes.' As you know from Chapter 6, this is what we call 'peeling back the layers of the onion'. We keep asking the question until the client has no more answers – they have nowhere else to go in terms of figuring out their reasons. Then we feel we've arrived at what we believe is the *real* issue; then the client has a far higher chance of succeeding.

If an overweight person was offered – guaranteed – £10,000 for every 10lb (4.5kg) of excess weight they lost (in fact, financial reward schemes do now exist as the global obesity battle gets ever more desperate), how many blocks of 10lb (4.5kg) would they lose? Our overweight client with 6 stone (38kg) to lose would collect a tax-free lump sum in excess of £80,000 if they reached their target weight.

Before you just pass over this scenario, rethink it for a minute. Would that *really* do it? Would that last, unsuccessful diet they undertook really have a different outcome? Could the real reason for their past failures be simply down to a lack of motivation? Did they want the positive outcome *enough*? Maybe they thought they did, but when it came down to it...

In the UK, there was an 18-year-old girl who had apparently tried a number of diets over a period of six years to lose 84lb (38kg) of excess weight; all had been unsuccessful. She was then selected to audition for a top TV talent show, and guess what – yep, you got it in one – when she appeared on TV five months later she was a perfect 135lb (61kg). So, what changed for her? Why did the diets that had proved to be unsuccessful suddenly work perfectly?

Be sure that you don't confuse motivation with willpower, though. It's different, and it must never be underrated. In a medical paper on the subject, William Miller Ph.D. talks of the similarity of food addiction to that of say, tobacco, stating that the route out of addiction involves finding more compelling alternatives.[1] We understand this to mean that the aforementioned 18-year-old girl found that the thought of appearing on national television was more appealing than burgers and fries.

For others, the motivation may come from a doctor telling them that the likelihood of their having a stroke is now off the scale, or that they've just joined the millions of people who have Type 2 diabetes.

IT'S ALWAYS YOUR CHOICE

You're sitting there now reading this and thinking that more than anything else in the world, you want to lose weight; you want to be slim. There's every reason under the sun to lose weight – marriage, sex, family, health issues, everything – so why not do it today? You see you *can* reach your target weight if you want to – maybe even this year, or by next summer. Deep down you *know* that. You can have a plate of profiteroles or a portion of chips, but understand this – you cannot *repeatedly* have both and expect to lose weight. Which is more important – the food or shifting the weight? Which do you want more?

Bad Eating Habits

Habit-forming in the field of hunger usually starts in childhood. We seldom ask our children whether they are hungry or not. We just say, 'It's 6 o'clock, come and have your dinner, and by the way, don't even think about leaving the table until you've cleared your plate.' Lesson one.

Often, this overfeeding – some would say force-feeding – is taken even further and children are encouraged to finish their food so they can be 'rewarded' with yet more food in the form of a sugar-laden dessert. What exactly is the logic behind that idea? Eat as much as you can and the prize is… more food!

Children are so often persuaded to eat by parents who don't understand the idea of true hunger. How about allowing them to eat small, kid-sized meals – taking what they want off a plate and nothing more. Don't make them finish it if they say they're full? Then they won't become conditioned in the way their parents were, and they'll know it's not a crime to leave food on a plate if you've had enough. Their stomachs won't become permanently stretched, either.

We've all seen something like this: the kids are playing in the garden when mum calls out, 'Come in for your dinner.' The kids respond with, 'Yes, coming in a minute,' as they jump in and out of a paddling pool, or bounce on a trampoline. Ten minutes later, mum urges them to come in because it's getting cold. 'Yes, we're coming…' they say. Half an hour later she has to go into the garden to drag them in – because they're having fun, doing great things. Food gets in the way. What could be more boring than sitting at a table and having to stuff your face with food you're not sure you even want?

It's interesting to think about how, or when, that situation actually changes in our lives, because it does – for many adults, going out to lunch or dinner is their number-one pastime. It's hard to even consider socializing with friends or family without bringing food into the equation. When friends phone us and ask if we are free and that they'll pick us up at 7 p.m., we presume – as most people would – that we're going out to dinner.

If they arrived and said, 'Hi, we've booked a lane at the bowling alley,' or 'How about going for a nice walk?' or 'Shall we go for a country drive?' we would pass out! Society has programmed us – or we have done it to ourselves – to believe that entertaining must involve food.

> 'It seems that they gave me the willpower I never had before. I now walk for at least an hour a day. My husband is so proud of me and cannot believe how well I have done. Now when I wake in the morning I don't think, "What shall I eat today?" but "What shall I wear?" as I feel so much more confident in everything I put on.'
> **GMB** CLIENT SPAIN

Do You Know What Hunger Feels Like?

The question 'Are you *really* hungry?' is one that isn't asked often enough. When did *you* last go without food for long enough to check it out; to find out what hunger feels like? If you want to, you could try fasting for a day (unless you have diabetes or another medical condition that means you need to keep eating regularly), not forgetting to drink plenty of water. How long do you think it would take before you *really* know what hunger is?

Many overweight people have a fear of hunger. But it's okay to feel hungry – it's actually no big deal and you really don't have to eat the minute you start to feel hunger pangs. In fact, you'll notice that after a time the pangs eventually subside – it's not an emergency that needs to be dealt with immediately.

Ask anyone who's had to fast before going into hospital, or before a blood test, just how they felt. However did they manage to go for 12 or 24 hours without food? Surely it must be impossible?

What would really happen to you if you fasted for a day – other than losing weight? You'd maybe detox a little and give your stomach, bowel and colon a break. Other than that, probably nothing. If you decide to try a fast, write down how you feel as you do it, and maybe do it more than once, then you will stand a reasonable chance of learning to recognize just what true hunger really is.

Why Do We Eat Too Much?

Absolutely everything to do with eating – or anything else for that matter – starts with a thought. It could be prompted by seeing a TV advert for a luxury food store – everything made to sound and look very sexy, with a seductive voiceover, beautiful photography, a table laid with a red and gold cloth, candles, background music, and an open log fire…

But have you ever seen an ad like that featuring an overweight couple, perspiring and undoing the top button of their jeans as they eat? No, you won't have. The actors in food adverts are healthy and slender; they're never podgy. They'd probably tell you that they wouldn't touch the fat-laden food they're advertising with a bargepole. They only appear in the ad because they're paid a small fortune to do so.

But the question is often not just *why* we are eating – because eating in moderation is fine – but *why we are eating so much*. Let's compare overeaters to smokers. Smokers have a thousand reasons for *why* they smoke – they're bored, they're depressed, it relaxes them, or wakes them up in the morning, and they'll often tell you that they enjoy smoking. But do they *really* enjoy the hot smoke going into their lungs and the coughing? No. Do they enjoy what it does to the taste of their food? Do they enjoy the brown stuff on their tongue, the financial cost, and feeling more and more like an outcast?

There's a side issue here. Why smokers smoke is, to a large degree, psychological. It's the same with food. Why do you eat too much? Is it for the feeling you get when you've stuffed so much food in there's a stretched feeling in your stomach? Is it the lying awake at night with indigestion? Is it having to buy boring, unflattering clothes, or always feeling self-conscious on a beach? Is that what you really like? Not very likely – it's all part of a matrix.

At this point, don't say to yourself that the reason you eat is because you like the taste of food. Try sitting down alone, somewhere quiet, and putting a square of chocolate on your tongue. Don't chew or suck it: just leave it to melt by itself, slowly; it may take a few minutes. During the time it's melting, you'll experience all the wonderful tastes and experiences of the chocolate, both physically and psychologically.

So, what happens when, 30 seconds later, you put another square in your mouth? What experiences do you think you'll get the second time? The truth is that you'll not get many at all; you've had the 'hit' from the chocolate, it's over. If you eat slowly and mindfully, and appreciate the texture and taste of your food, you'll soon realize that quantity plays virtually no part at all.

Of course, the situation is not helped by the dramatic rise in 'all-inclusive holidays' of the 'eat and drink as much as you want' variety. On a recent flight we sat next to a couple who told us they were returning from holiday. When we asked if they'd enjoyed it, all they talked about for the next hour was the brilliant food, the massive portions, the midnight buffets; they even proudly showed us the undone buttons on their jeans — 'That's after just 10 days,' they said proudly. They'd already decided to return the following year. The accommodation, the flights, the weather, the places they'd visited didn't get a mention — we thought it was sad.

Distinguishing Want from Need

There's a basic bit of psychology connected with overeating — the same as with addiction. It's all about the confusion of two words: want and need. A simple trick is to try to remove the word 'want' from your vocabulary. From now on, stop asking yourself, or allowing others to ask you, if you *want* a cheeseburger or if you *want* a bar of chocolate; try instead to say, 'Do I *need* a...?' More often than not, you'll find that you need the burger or chocolate about as much as you need a heart attack.

Try it next time you decide to put something in your mouth. Stop for just a second, and then ask yourself the 'need' question — plus, of course, whether putting this in your mouth will move you closer to, or further away, from your goal weight.

Being able to identify when you've had enough to eat is a skill many overweight people have to learn from scratch. Our research/analysis of clients' data clearly shows a correlation between fast eating and being overweight. Overweight people eat as if the world is about to end. They're guaranteed to be the first at the table to finish, yet in the next breath they'll tell you how much they love food, and how much pleasure they gain from it. Which is quite strange, as fast eaters seldom gain the maximum pleasure from food, or indeed eating.

You see when you eat quickly, your 10,000 taste buds[2] – most of which are on your tongue – and the olfactory receptors in your nose don't get the chance to inform your brain about all the wonderful tastes in your mouth. If you chew slowly, not only do you get to distinguish the different tastes, but the chemicals released travel up your nose, allowing you to gain additional pleasure and satisfaction. That's why taste is experienced less when you have a cold, or indeed when you smoke.

If a washing machine won't work as well as it should when it's overfilled, why expect your stomach to be any different?

Of course, once you've swallowed the food the experience has passed. Once it's passed to your throat you may as well have been eating tissue paper for all you've actually appreciated it, so if you're eating something you enjoy, eat it slowly, and chew it thoroughly. Keep it in your mouth for as long as possible. Of course, if it's a foul-tasting medicine knock it back quickly!

For an overweight person who eats quickly, the new skill of eating slowly and enjoying their food can take a little time to master, as their poor stretched stomach doesn't have time to tell the brain it doesn't need any more, it's had enough food. Furthermore, if they weren't actually hungry when they sat down to eat, the signals to the brain will be totally confused. It's the same when people eat for emotional reasons: they might be eating continually, but they never feel full. Ice cream doesn't overcome boredom, or loneliness; food will never solve the emotional reasons for eating.

THE TWO TYPES OF MEAL

We believe that meals can be divided into two kinds: those that matter and those that don't. The two evening meals on Friday and Saturday, say, might be special for you – whether you're at home with your partner or eating out. They can still be healthy, but you might decide to have a bottle of wine, or a dessert, and spoil yourselves.

The meals you eat on the other five nights of the week are just not quite as important. They could be simple meals such as scrambled egg on toast, or a basic salad. They're not special. You'll eat 1,000 meals a year on average, so if you get it wrong or relax your regime for 50 meals, that's about a meal every week, and it'll be nigh on impossible to undo the good you've done with the other 950.

One question we ask which often starts an interesting conversation is, 'What are the disadvantages of doing a particular thing and getting to your goal weight?' People usually answer very quickly, saying they believe there aren't any disadvantages. Often that's just not true, though, and the situation it highlights is the downfall of many dieters. They often under-appreciate the pull of the Friday night curry with friends, say, or the socializing down the pub, the gut-busting Sunday lunch. There are always downsides, and there's always a price to pay.

When Do You Stop Eating?

Take a few moments to think about this question. Then imagine you're in a restaurant, your meal in front of you, knife and fork in your hands... when will you finish? The truth is that, like most overweight people, you'll usually stop when the plate is empty. But how can that work? When the waiter took your order, the chef didn't come out to see whether you are male or female, need less food, had a heavy lunch today; he doesn't know if you have a large or a small frame. In fact, the person providing your calorie intake doesn't know anything about you at all, which is potentially very dangerous.

Of course, none of this matters to people who don't have 'a problem' with their weight; they automatically stop eating before they even feel full. Overweight people tend to hoover their way through the plate until it's empty. Next time you go out to dinner, watch. Be discreet, but observe. You'll quickly see that people are simply not aware of why they stop eating at the end of a meal.

They stop eating when the plate's empty and not before, and if they save their favourite food to the end, the problem is even worse. If the portion size is too big – and they usually are – they're in trouble. When we ask people how long they think the pleasure of a plate of chips will last, they answer, quite accurately, 15 minutes or less; how long would the pleasure of being at *your* target weight last?

**If you leave your favourite food until last,
it guarantees that you'll eat everything else
on your plate.**

The final part of this equation is that the overweight person's definition of feeling full is often totally different from a slim person's. They'll have a big meal but they won't feel they've eaten enough until they feel fit to burst. They actually *enjoy* that feeling of being really stuffed full. Or at least they think they do.

Food is fuel for your body and gives you energy, so, ideally, after you've finished eating a meal you should feel energized. If you feel as if you need to lie around and sleep it off, then you've seriously overeaten and all your energy is being taken up by your poor digestive system working hard to process all that extra food.

Imagine going for a brisk walk *before* you eat a meal; consider how comfortable you would feel doing that. Then think what it would be like *after* a meal to get up and do that same walk again; you should be able to do it without feeling desperately uncomfortable. That's the level of fullness you're aiming at. Often, a big person will eat until they can't even move off the chair, never mind go for a walk. That is way, way too much.

THE 'FULLNESS' SCALE

If you've eaten the perfect quantity at a meal, you should get up from the table just having had enough. If you get up and go, phewwww, that's not good. Try finishing when you're no more than 80 per cent full. We have a scale of fullness to help you learn not to eat too much. It's a good idea to keep a notebook to jot down how you feel when you've eaten the following: a couple of forkfuls; then a couple more; then a third of your plate; then half; and so on.

As you eat, mark yourself out of 10 on a 'scale of fullness'. Once you've got the hang of this, the idea is to stop eating when you're no more than 6 or 7 out of 10. It's too easy to think you're hungry if you haven't tested your own levels of hunger/fullness.

Going There First

Instead of just thinking, wondering and dreaming about all the things that are going to happen between now and the time when you've got down to the weight and size you want to be, try taking some time out *and go there now*.

Find somewhere quiet, where you can really relax and daydream. Close your eyes and use a bit of visualization to go to that place and see what it's like. See yourself at your ideal size. Really *see* it and *feel* it. What do you smell like? (Yes, *smell* like). How much energy do you have? What about your level of confidence – are people around you interacting with you differently now that you're at your perfect weight?

Live it all out in your mind. What's buying clothes going to feel like? Which shops will you go into? Will you still have to avoid public changing rooms? What's sex going to be like? What will it be like to be able to put the tray down in front of you on your next holiday flight, and see the strange little space between your belly and the tray? To feel confident that you won't need a seat belt extension ever again?

Visualizing how you will feel when you reach your goal weight is an important weapon in your GMB armoury. Next time you're dining out and you're not sure whether to have a starter or not, try to see the 'new you'; take a moment to remember how good you're going to look and feel. Think about your renewed energy and your new level of confidence. You'll have those positive feelings for the rest of your life – it's called 'going there first'.

Alternatively, you can choose to have that starter, which you probably don't need, and just get a little bit fatter. You decide.

When Martin started the GMB therapy he made a simple promise to himself: every Monday he would weigh a bit less than the previous Monday. It mattered little whether it was 2lb (900g) or 2oz (57g), as long as it was going down. Every Monday was a celebration.

Try, Could and Should

People who are determined not to succeed automatically pre-programme themselves with what we call 'licence to fail' words – words like try, should and could. These words are just cop-outs; they don't mean anything. They're losers' words. There's no commitment, no determination, and it sounds as though the outcome is already decided: 'Oh, I'm going to *try* to do it, but it might not actually work,' or 'I *should* be able to do it,' and so on.

If you put this book down now, are you going to eat 500 fewer calories than you need every day for the next week and lose a pound (0.45kg), or are you going to get fatter? If you ask yourself that and the answer is 'I'm going to try,' don't bother, because you're not determined or fully convinced enough to do it yet!

Can you stick to something for a month? If you say, 'I should be able to,' or 'I could do,' how would you analyse those statements? The question asks for a straightforward yes or no. Not a could, or a should or a try.

Is it going to work for you – everything you've read so far in the book? All the planning, answering the questionnaire, learning about your bad food habits? If your answer is, 'You know what, I'm really going to give this a try,' you're obviously setting yourself up to just go out and have a burger and chips. What does 'try' mean? The question is: 'Are you going to succeed? Yes or no?' It's a cop-out to say that you'll try, or you should be able to do it.

Will you do it, yes or no? If you're still using the word try, some part of your motivation to succeed is missing. Start to analyse the internal dialogue you have: start to look for the coulds, shoulds and tries.

> *'To eat is a necessity, but to eat intelligently is an art.'*
> La Rochefoucauld

Beware the Diet Terrorists

Do you know any terrorists? Of course not, you cry. Well, we bet you do! We believe that those friends and family who invite you to dinner and feed you four courses – plus nibbles to start with, wine with every course, cheese after, chocolates with the coffee – are Diet Terrorists who cause chaos with your food choices. Terrorists and chaos are just words we use to identify people who screw up your eating habits. Who's going to set *you* up?

The Diet Terrorists are clever. They can, and often do, take on many guises. They can even disguise themselves as situations or events. Once, Martin realized before a flight that he'd forgotten his glasses, just as an announcement came over the tannoy saying his flight was delayed. He now had three hours to kill. He was alone, with no reading glasses, and at that moment he was sitting outside a bar that served drinks and snacks. In that instance, the Diet Terrorists won.

If you think a dinner party you went to was a disaster because you overate, stop and ask yourself whether you were there as a guest or as a prisoner? Did your hosts *force* you to eat? Couldn't you have said no? Would they have stopped being friends with you because you turned down their pudding? Would they have shunned you for not having seconds? Are they friends or just an excuse to get fat?

You go to friends for dinner and they load you up with alcohol, peanuts, pickles, hors d'oeuvres, canapés, crisps – all this food before you're even seated at the table. You haven't had the first course and you've undone a notch on your belt. Then they come to your home, and of course, guess what happens – you produce twice as much, twice as fancy. The competition sets in. You put out a huge bowl of peanuts yet you top it up before it goes down too far; there's also a big jug of dip – you're scared you're not going to have enough – laden with cholesterol, a recipe for a heart attack.

> ***Everything starts as a thought.***
> ***Barely anything can happen in your***
> ***body without it starting as a thought.***

You're in the deli section of the supermarket when you see a roast chicken on a spit. Maybe it reminds you of family picnics or barbecues. Thought creates desire, and then action. The action could be to buy a packet of cooked chicken drumsticks, or it could be to walk past the chicken and enjoy the moment. But, as long as you are aware that everything starts with a thought, and how that process is going to run, you'll be okay.

People often say that they're fine as long as they don't go out with a particular friend with whom they always go to the same place and have the same foods. Identify for yourself who your Diet Terrorists are – and the places and things that combine with them to give you food-choice headaches – and work out some avoidance techniques.

Perhaps, if you are having a particularly healthy week, you could go to a Japanese restaurant rather than an Italian one, or make it a week when you don't see the friend who loves to have a couple of bottles of red wine.

We have another theory – maybe fat people *think* too slowly. Maybe normal-weight people are faster thinkers. At a party, waiters are coming round with sausage rolls. *Full of fat, no taste, don't want one*, the thin people think and ignore them.

Maybe the fat people aren't quite there yet, though: they have one and think *afterwards* (probably regretting their decision). Maybe fat people haven't yet learned to walk away for five minutes and work out what to do if they're faced with a food choice they're finding hard. They could press Pause… you'll learn how in just a few pages.

PAIN NOW, PLEASURE LATER

It doesn't matter which way you describe it, weight loss is a process in which you *cannot* see the immediate changes that you might (illogically and unrealistically) be hoping for. The 'pain' of changing your food habits inevitably comes some time before you experience the 'pleasure', or 'gain' of better health – smaller clothes sizes, more energy and so on. However, with GMB, you need never again feel quite as despondent, quite as negative, about your appearance as you do at the start of your weight-loss journey. With every week that passes, every pound/kg lost, you'll be feeling progressively more positive.

Learning New Habits

Much of what lies behind the Gastric Mind Band is to do with getting rid of your existing bad food habits and replacing them with new, healthier ones. Habits and skills can be learned a lot quicker if they're attractive enough to you. It might take 21 days to learn a new habit, or it might take six weeks; it could be even take as long as eight months.[3] It's down to motivation.

Let's say you find it hard to remember phone numbers. Then you meet a stunning girl in the street, or a guy in the frozen food section at the supermarket, and they tell you their phone number. Lo and behold you remember it! If something is positive, it's easy to learn quickly. The things you don't want to do, you find harder to pick up.

We 'unlearn' bad habits and learn new ones via the neural pathways in our brain, which carry the signals. You can imagine these as a physical path you're going to walk along; when it's a new habit the path might be narrow, and it'll be hard to find your way through the weeds. This is how you'll feel when learning to eat less – learning not to reach for a doughnut or a curry.

You'll have to work quite hard to make your own pathway through. But the more often you do this action, this habit or behaviour, the more you'll make the path wider and the route easier. In the end, it'll be like an elevated three-lane highway.

This is exactly the way that the signals and pathways work in the brain. New habits that you're only just starting on are not that strong in your mind, but once you've repeated them enough times you'll do the behaviour almost on autopilot.

Which is, of course, what you've done with your current eating habits. Eating for the wrong reasons is so ingrained that it's something you do automatically. In order to change these habits – to create new ones and leave the old ones behind – you have to create new neural pathways, just like the path through the undergrowth.

Bad programming = bad habits

The new pathways will be a bit harder to follow to begin with, but you'll trample them down and eventually they'll disappear completely and you'll only be able to go down the new ones. Once you've created the new habits there's no reason to go back to the old ones. However, if it does happen, see it as what it is — a lapse, not a *relapse*. Learn from your mistakes, take knowledge from them.

Habits such as walking, talking, driving, shaving, etc. are created for us to make our lives easier. If you had to relearn how to clean your teeth on a daily basis life would become a chore and it would all take a very long time. When you're starting on a new habit, you have to consciously make the effort to do this behaviour, whatever it is.

Initially, it will feel unnatural. Driving a car, walking, talking, riding a bike — you have to do these things over and over again, and eventually, when you've done them often enough, you get to the point where your conscious mind doesn't need to concentrate on them any more and that's when your subconscious mind takes over.

The subconscious mind doesn't recognize logic at all — it can't distinguish good habits from bad ones. All it does is what it's programmed to do. It's like a computer in that it takes in all the information we give it, and then churns it out exactly as it's been programmed to do. If you've programmed your subconscious in such a way that every time you're stressed you reach for a bar of chocolate, it will throw out that behaviour every time you're in a stressful situation because it thinks it's helping you. Once you've repeated the behaviour often enough, it becomes strongly ingrained in your subconscious mind.

If there's ever a conflict between your conscious and your subconscious minds, such as happens when you're trying to break a habit, the much more powerful subconscious mind will always win in the end, eventually causing you to go back to whatever habits (including eating habits) it considers are 'normal' for you.

In order to make permanent changes in your life, then, it's necessary to get your subconscious in agreement with what you want to accomplish *consciously* – rather than fighting and struggling to work against it. This is why diets – which rely solely on 'willpower' and the use of your conscious mind – are very rarely successful. It has nothing to do with being weak-willed, it's just a perfect demonstration of how powerful the human mind is.

It's getting the subconscious to grasp the severity of the motivation, to see it as real.

DOES WILLPOWER ACTUALLY EXIST?

There are people who say that willpower is just a word we use when we haven't got another explanation for why we can't do something. It's arguable, they say, that it exists. How would *you* define willpower? Is it doing something you *don't want* to do? Or is it stopping yourself from doing something you *want* to do?

Choosing the Right Body Fuel

Picture yourself as the sort of car you'd love to own – your pride and joy. Your body is the vehicle that takes you on your journey through life, so you ought to treat it with the same respect as you treat your car, if not more. After all, when your car wears out, you can always buy another one, but you only have one body to get you through the whole of your life. If your car runs on petrol, you wouldn't dream of filling it with diesel instead, because you know the engine is designed to use petrol.

That said, although we say you can eat less healthily occasionally – no more than one day a week at most – strangely (with very few exceptions depending on make/model), the same applies to the fuel in a car. You can actually get it wrong – put diesel in a petrol car or vice versa – and, providing the quantity of the wrong fuel is no more than 5–10 per cent, you'll do no lasting harm.[4] You'll need to get back to the right fuel as soon as you possibly can though. This is remarkably similar to eating the 'wrong' foods, wouldn't you say?

In the same way, you are aware that your body functions best when you eat healthy, nutritious foods, so you shouldn't expect to be able to consume large quantities of highly processed, unnatural foods (of poor nutritional value) and still maintain a healthy weight.

Continuing with the car analogy, your vehicle's fuel tank has a warning buzzer or a light, or at least a basic gauge, to let you know when it's close to empty, and this serves as a reminder for you to fill up. In a similar way, your body sends out hunger pangs as a signal that your stomach is empty, and this is your reminder to 'refuel' (i.e. eat). It wouldn't occur to you to pull in at every service station you pass just to try and squeeze some more fuel into the tank, so why would you do this with your body?

You'd think it was wasteful to allow excess fuel to spill out all over the petrol station forecourt, yet overweight people are doing a similar thing with their own bodies when they eat excess food for emotional reasons rather than to satisfy real hunger.

Identifying Your Triggers

You've already identified your own motivation for change. Now you must acknowledge what triggers you to eat, and how simply recognizing this is your first step to dealing with the same situation differently next time. Our emotional and behavioural triggers for eating are many and varied, as the chart below shows.

Emotional/Behavioural triggers	Physical triggers
Smelling food and seeing food	The only natural trigger we should respond to is hunger
Seeing someone eating food	
Being offered some food	
Reading a recipe in a magazine	
Seeing a food advert on TV or watching a food programme	
Reading a description of a banquet in a historical novel	
Filling the car with fuel, going into a shop	
Going to a newsagent and automatically buying sweets	
Travelling to and from work – having a snack habit	
Walking into the kitchen and opening the fridge door	
Boredom and stress	

Emotional/Behavioural triggers	Physical triggers
Having a hard day at work	
Feeling upset or annoyed	
Depression	
Loneliness	
Celebrations	

Did you pay attention to the length of the two lists?

Having experienced a trigger, you have a thought that leads you to desire or crave food and you make the decision to eat. If you're not hungry this is, of course, totally illogical. CBT teaches us how to recognize the sabotaging thoughts that lead to inappropriate eating, and turn them into more helpful thoughts instead.

Everyone is exposed to exactly the same triggers, but slim people respond differently to them, and tend only to eat in response to physical hunger. For example, if a slim person passes by a baker's not long after eating they will certainly appreciate the lovely smell of freshly baked bread, but it wouldn't occur to them to go inside the shop and buy something to eat there and then; after all, they think, *I only had lunch an hour ago.*

On the other hand, if you put a person who tends to struggle with their weight in the same situation, they'll probably be in the shop in a flash, buying bread and croissants, and maybe a cream cake too, as they think that because they've caught a whiff of something tasty they 'can't possibly resist it and absolutely have to have it', despite having eaten a meal just an hour earlier.

'Instead of seeing food as "the enemy" I've learned to enjoy and savour the food that I like eating and balance my intake in a healthy way. I eat more slowly, have less on my plate, and recognize much faster when I've eaten enough to satisfy my hunger, and stop.

'Chocolate has always been my favourite comfort food and I do still give in to it every now and then. However, once I have it out of my system, I forgive myself, put it behind me and get back with the programme. I've reduced my weight by five stone (32kg) in the past year and I'm still losing!'
GMB CLIENT **C.T.**

How to Handle Your Triggers

In her book *The Beck Diet Solution,* US psychologist Dr Judith Beck (daughter of CBT founder Dr Aaron Beck) gives a helpful description to convey the idea of the two different ways of reacting to these triggers. She identifies two psychological 'muscles' – the 'resistance muscle' and the 'giving in' muscle.[5]

If you always eat in response to triggers, you're establishing a certain pattern of behaviour – strengthening your 'giving in' muscle – but if you recognize that triggers are not commands that have to be obeyed, and you resist the temptation to eat unnecessarily, you are establishing a more positive and helpful pattern of behaviour, or strengthening your 'resistance muscle'. The more often you repeat a certain action, the easier it is for that behaviour to become a natural reaction for you.

People with weight problems often share certain traits that can sabotage their efforts to shed excess weight. Among these are:

- Eating when not hungry.

- Eating for emotional reasons rather than simple hunger.

- Deluding themselves about how much they eat.

- Eating to the point of being stuffed full rather than comfortably satisfied.

- Eating quickly and not recognizing when they are satisfied.

- Skipping breakfast or other meals.

- Not 'being able' to leave food on their plate.

- Putting themselves under too much pressure about what they're eating, and blowing 'lapses' out of proportion.

- Having unrealistic expectations. How long did it take them to get that fat? How can it be lost overnight?

- Feeling that life is unfair on them when their slim friends seem to be able to eat whatever they want. Not recognizing that the slim person will have been compensating in the day(s) before and after eating a big meal.

Distorting the Truth

CBT has identified a number of 'Cognitive Distortions' – the ways in which our mind convinces us to believe things that aren't true. First defined by Dr Aaron Beck, the more common examples were then made more popular by David D Burns, Judith Beck and others. Using some of their labels, here's our own look at how you are probably viewing your problems with food and eating.

Perfectionism, or All or Nothing Thinking

You have a really good week, food-wise – getting through Monday, Tuesday and Wednesday eating mindfully, staying on track. On Thursday you're tempted to eat something you don't need. Let's say a biscuit. You eat it, and straight away you think that one biscuit is a disaster, a catastrophe. It's undone everything you've achieved this week. You believe the logical thing to do is then to eat the whole pack of biscuits because that *one* biscuit has already done the damage anyway.

The CBT way of viewing such a situation is to put it in perspective. See the biscuit as a lapse, a hiccup. Get yourself back on track right now. Be focused and mindful of what you eat for the rest of the day, and then Thursday will still have been a good day. Maybe not perfect, but that's realistic and acceptable. You're not aiming to be perfect, because we're all human and perfection simply doesn't exist.

Of course, some people will take it to the extreme, thinking that it's almost the weekend so they might as well allow themselves to lose the plot for the next few days and promise themselves to get back on track on Monday. All diets start on a Monday, after all! But it's always easier to get back on track *now*, rather than leaving it until Monday. Remember, that one biscuit doesn't constitute a disaster – it's how you react to the situation that will either create or avoid a disastrous outcome.

Discounting the Positive

A classic example of this is when you get on the scales, find that you're a pound (0.45kg) lighter than last time you weighed yourself, and yet your reaction is, 'Oh, is that all!? I still have X number of pounds, kilos, stones, to get rid of before I can even *start* to feel good about myself.' So many people do this. With CBT you recognize that you're that much closer to where you want to be. It's a small step in the right direction, which is all that matters. Celebrate your achievement, rather than focusing on the negative and thinking about what's still ahead of you.

Jumping to Conclusions

This is what happens when, as you walk into a party and several people turn around to look at you, you think they're judging you, noticing what you're wearing, thinking critical thoughts, labelling you as fat and ugly. In fact, you're just *assuming* you know what other people are thinking about you, and tending to think it's something negative. This is directly related to how you think about yourself. You're self-critical. In fact, those people are just mildly curious because they heard the sound of an opening door. Most people are caught up in their own lives and aren't spending their whole time thinking critically about others.

Fortune Telling

This is a variation of Jumping to Conclusions. It means predicting how things will turn out based on what's happened in the past, and usually putting a negative slant on things. For example, you say, 'I've tried various diets and nothing has worked as a long-term solution, so why is this time going to be any different? It's not going to work, I'm going to fail, so why am I even trying in the first place?'

CBT teaches you to recognize that what's happened in the past is gone. We can't change the past, but we can learn from past mistakes and where things went wrong, and then draw a line under the past and concentrate on the present – which we *can* do something about. It's true that if you keep doing the same thing you've always done, of course you'll get the same result, but the fact is you don't *have* to do the same thing. You can actually change how you react, and get a different, more positive result – the one you want.

Emotional Reasoning

If, when you justify eating something, you apportion the reason, or 'blame', on an emotion, there is clearly no logic to that. For example, you might think (or say), 'I've had a really hard day at work, so I deserve to eat a bar of chocolate,' or 'I've had a row with my best friend and I'm going to cheer myself up with a tub of ice cream.'

The CBT way of looking at things is to recognize that the only problem food solves is hunger. So if hunger isn't the problem in the first place, food will never be the solution in any of these situations. All the food is doing is providing a temporary distraction from the real problem, and far from helping to solve the problem, it actually exacerbates it.

Self-Deluding Thinking

If you eat something in secret and no one sees you, or if you eat standing up, do you convince yourself that this doesn't count? Maybe you believe that there aren't any calories in broken biscuits (yes, some people really convince themselves of this!). The CBT viewpoint would say you should be logical, and take responsibility. All the food and drink you put in your mouth counts, regardless of where you are, who you're with, or who has seen you.

Confusing Want with Need

We looked at this earlier in the chapter. An example would be seeing some food in front of you and convincing yourself that, because you like the look of it and *want* to eat it, this automatically means you must *need* it. The CBT take on this is simple: wanting something and needing something are two completely separate things. You need to ask yourself the right question in order to get the appropriate answer. Don't ask yourself, 'Do I *want* to eat this food?' – your answer will almost certainly be 'Yes!' – instead ask yourself, 'Do I *need* to eat this food?' In other words, 'Am I actually, physically hungry?'

One way of dealing with Cognitive Distortions is to visualize yourself standing in court, presenting your 'case' to a judge and jury. What evidence do you have that what you're thinking makes sense? Would another person, on hearing your story, say you were totally right or completely crazy to think that way? Is there a different way of looking at it? Would your case be thrown out of court?

Of course, you could also ask yourself, 'What would I advise a friend if they were saying the same thing to me?' Your answer might be interesting. It's always easier to think logically about other people's problems and give sound advice to them!

Think Before You Act

You may be one of those people who say they don't have a chance to stop themselves before putting food in their mouth – it's in before they've realized it. But, there's *always* that split second between having the thought and going ahead with the action. That's because, as we've said before, *everything starts with an idea, a thought.* It might only be a split second, but it's a thought that passes through your mind, and then you react to it.

Your thought might be, 'I'm feeling upset', or 'I've got a few minutes to fill', or 'I fancy one of those biscuits.' Nothing to do with hunger. It's a thought relating simply to the food being there, or to the emotion of wanting to feel better and associating that with food. It gets to the point where you're not actually noticing the thought itself – you think you're reaching for the food and simply can't stop yourself. But if you put the whole episode into slow motion, you'll realize the thought *is* there. The key is to recognize it and then stop yourself from acting on it by not following through and putting the food in your mouth.

You can make it a comedy moment in your mind if it helps – a long, drawn-out slow-motion STTOOOOPPPP!!!!

KAY LINDLEY'S STORY

When Kay Lindley, a primary school head teacher, started with GMB, she weighed 22 stone 10lb (144.5kg) and wore size 32 clothes. She was very clear about what was needed to fix her weight problem. 'When I lost weight in the past,' she says, 'it seemed as though a switch had flicked in my brain which made me able to restrict food intake, but over which I had no control. It had operated totally independently from my conscious thinking. I needed it to be "magically" activated!'

Kay – a twice-divorced mother of one – has had a weight problem all her life; her mother and aunts also struggled with 'pear-shape' weight issues. She considered gastric band surgery but discounted it mainly on the grounds of cost. 'GMB seemed like a possible alternative,' she says. 'I decided against surgery when I heard exactly what was involved in the surgical option.'

Now 7½ stone (48kg) lighter, Kay is happy to explain her weight history. First, though, we should let her give us an insight into her own wry way of looking at things:

'Right, let's get this straight from the beginning: I was a big baby at more than 10½lb (4.7kg). Okay, so that was 60 years ago, but it's my excuse and I'm sticking to it. I have plenty of other excuses too. Everyone in my mother's family has the same big bone structure, and all are pear shaped. It's in the genes and it can't be changed. My mother was a domestic science teacher and most of her classes were about cakes and their decoration – coffee cream, chocolate icing, jam fillings – need I say more?

'Just after the war, with children starving around the world, it was almost criminal to leave food uneaten on your plate. How dare you disrespect the poor starving children in this way? You see, being obese isn't my fault. It's beyond my control and I'm the innocent victim of this conspiracy!'

Kay has lost a lot of weight in the past – she dropped 7 stone (44.5kg) on one occasion and 4–5 stone (25–32kg) on another; in both cases she ate a highly restricted and repetitive diet – e.g. a jacket potato with tuna mayonnaise for dinner every day!

She tried many diet programmes, including Weight Watchers, but always replaced anything lost and more when she returned to her previous eating patterns. 'I didn't eat because I was hungry,' she says, 'I ate as a treat, a reward, a comfort and so on. I didn't think that stopping eating when I felt full was going to work, as I'd always felt full but kept on eating anyway, and this seemed to be normal.' Kay convinced herself that if she hadn't enjoyed eating something its calories didn't count and she could have something else to take away the taste.

Turning Things Around with GMB
A Type 2 diabetic with arthritis in one hip, both knees and both hands, Kay's peak weight was 24 stone (152.7kg).

Her goal with GMB? To be fit and active enough to go travelling, as well as to walk around the school where she works without experiencing so much pain. 'I hoped that GMB would "flick the switch" for me, and it seems to have done so,' she says. 'I started to lose weight in the very first week, and a month later I'd lost 26lb (12kg). Overall, I lost 5½ stone (35kg) in the first 7½ months.

'I went on a study tour to China – an exhausting experience which involved walking long distances and climbing lots of stairs. It was hard going, but I did everything, including a visit to the Great Wall, and I wouldn't have been able to do any of it had I not lost a good deal of weight before I went. I was tired of seeing myself as a victim – someone who couldn't do things rather than someone who could. Mobility was a clear daily example of this.

'I haven't even considered overriding the GMB,' Kay says matter-of-factly. 'I did have wine while I was in China, which I don't usually have. I used to drink a bottle of wine a day, but I'm now on a no-alcohol regime unless I'm in a social situation such as our staff Christmas dinner.

'For me the most significant aspect of the whole treatment was the CBT. None of what we discussed was new to me, but spending the time focusing on me and my thoughts was a luxury I rarely have. I knew very clearly all the things I was doing wrongly and had been for many years. After losing weight, I tended to treat myself because I had been so good! Before long I was eating easily as much as before, if not more. However, bringing all that thinking together, and spending time focusing on my bad habits, made a bigger impact than ever before.

'I've had a reduction in my diabetic medication because my sugar levels have regularly been much lower than before. I couldn't wait to get on the scales. When I did and Marion announced I'd lost a staggering five stone (32kg), it was hugs all round.

'This is still work in progress,' Kay concludes. 'So far the progress has been very, very good and long may it continue. Having lost 7½ stone (48kg), I felt comfortable with the weight I had achieved and my current aim is to maintain this weight. I may decide, in the future, to lose some more, but for now I am happy.

'My diabetes is fully under control. I'm now on the lowest doses of the tablets for the condition and only need to be reviewed annually by the nurse rather than every three months by the specialist doctor.

'It's a great buzz to pick up a pair of trousers or a T-shirt and know they will fit. I sold all my big clothes, which raised £30 to go towards the new items. It's win, win! Remember, I had nearly 60 years of hard practice in becoming obese. If GMB can work for me then I think it can work for anyone.'

Kay has been featured on UK television's GMTV and in many daily newspapers and magazines in the UK, which were keen to cover her remarkable story.

Chapter 11
Pause Button Therapy

When it comes to ill-judged choices and snap decisions, people who are struggling to overcome a weight problem are up there with the worst. How many times have you eaten biscuit after biscuit, loving them all, and then five minutes later you regret the first more than anything? How many times have you beaten yourself up after drinking that second or third glass of wine, which is doing anything but helping your fight with excess fat?

Through our work at the clinic, it became clear to us that if there was a way of freezing time and enabling people to get into a 'safe zone' – freeing them up to consider the consequences of their actions – they would find it so much easier to think things through and reach better decisions.

Pause Button Therapy® (PBT) is that safe zone. Use it and use it: make it your best friend and this tool will help you stop yourself 'in the act' and recognize the better choice you can make if you just give yourself some thinking time.

Marion says that she can't honestly remember *how* she came up with a progression to a mental remote control device, but that's exactly what she did. 'I not only wanted people to stop themselves "in the act", but to pursue the idea so they could see themselves in five minutes' time *after* eating a bar of chocolate, *and also* see themselves in five minutes' time having *not* eaten it so they could compare the consequences of their actions,' she says.

'Because I thought it was important to strengthen clients' experience of the two options they were weighing up, I was imagining it visually, and the idea seemed so like using a TV remote that I kept thinking about the possibilities. Martin and I brainstormed and tweaked, and figured out ways to incorporate all the main remote control buttons, and that's how PBT was born!'

If you have Low Frustration Tolerance to a particular food, or smell of food, all your other logic, control, self-discipline, goes out of the window. It's as if this thing has some sort of a hold over you – it's consuming your whole being and turning you into a quivering wreck – and you even feel that if you don't go ahead and give in to it then you will literally just about collapse in a heap and die. (Does this sound familiar at all?)

The way out of this situation, out of the 'I can't stand this any longer' feeling, is to escape – and sadly, in the case of food, that means to *eat it*! Somehow you convince yourself that at that moment in time the 'advantages' of eating right there and then outweigh the 'disadvantages' of not eating in order to weigh a bit less some time in the future.

How to Use Your Pause Button

Whenever you find yourself in this – seemingly hopeless – situation, it's the perfect time to employ the Pause Button. All you need to do is imagine that you have a remote control for your life (similar to the one you use for your DVD player, etc.), so you can pause/fast-forward/rewind and so on as and when necessary.

First, picture yourself in a situation in which your greatest weakness (chocolate, crisps, biscuits, whatever it is) is sitting there right in front of you and you are starting to feel weak and about to reach out and gulp it down on the spot.

Take a deep breath and say to yourself, 'stop'. Then put yourself on 'Pause' by pressing your Pause Button to physically freeze-frame yourself. Now, while you are on Pause, spend the next few seconds running through the whole scenario in your mind as if watching a film of yourself – like using a DVD player. See yourself going ahead and eating whatever it is that you're feeling tempted by, and enjoying (or maybe not even enjoying!) a few quick seconds of gratification from it.

Then, in your mind, Fast-Forward to five minutes *after* you've finished eating, press Play and concentrate now on how you are feeling and what you're thinking. We bet you're going through the usual routine of feeling guilty and beating yourself up – telling yourself you've been stupid for scoffing all of that unnecessary food: 'Why on earth have I done this to myself yet again when I promised myself I wouldn't?' and so on.

Pause Button Therapy is a really effective technique you can use when you are feeling tempted to eat something that you know full well you don't actually need.

So, now you've reminded yourself of exactly how bad you're going to feel if you *do* go ahead and eat the tempting food, you can mentally Rewind back to the present – remembering that you're still on Pause physically – and run through the scenario once more. This time, though – because you're the director of this movie of your life and are in control of the scenes – you're going to add in the nice, 'happy ever after' ending.

This time you see yourself recognizing that you're not actually hungry and you certainly don't need that food, no matter how much you think you want it. It's just a desire or a craving – one of those sabotaging thoughts that you need to squash immediately, not a command that absolutely must be obeyed.

See yourself deciding to walk away from the food and distracting yourself in some way by reading a book, calling a friend, etc., and then Fast-Forward to five minutes afterwards. What are you thinking and how are you feeling now? You are going to be feeling so virtuous, strong and positive, so proud of yourself, because you know that you've reacted in the most positive way and have done the right thing at last! Ideally, choosing the 'happy ever after' ending will seem much more appealing and attractive than going down the same old road and repeatedly making the same mistakes.

In the end a thought can only take up as much space in your head as you allow it to, so if you recognize a sabotaging thought as such, you have the power and control to stop it in its tracks right there and then if you want to. Or you can choose to allow it to build up out of all proportion. So, the outcome is really your own choice.

PBT Puts You in Control

No one ever holds you down and physically forces food into your mouth. And food can't magically leap off the table and throw itself down your throat. It certainly doesn't have any special powers. It can't talk to you – no matter how much you 'hear' it calling out your name. It's actually just a pile of inert ingredients; how can it have any control over you, an intelligent human being?

Notice how we use the words 'power', 'control' and 'choice' here – PBT is all about empowerment and getting you to recognize that *you* are the one in control, and you can decide what the outcome will be, depending on how you react to a situation or stimulus.

Now you can mentally Rewind back to the present. You have just shown yourself the possible options and two totally different outcomes to this situation, and it's up to you to choose the path you're going to take. Before doing anything else, take a moment longer to find your list of reasons why it's so important to you to be slimmer.

Ask yourself right now what's more important to you – going for that instant gratification of eating the food, or the long-term benefits of being slimmer? The truth is that you can't choose both. You can't continue eating all that unnecessary food *and* choose to be slimmer than you are now.

The next step is to take yourself off Pause and make your choice – are you going to go down that same old road by eating unnecessary food and putting up with all the negative consequences that follow, or are you going to take a more positive route and not eat the food, which will mean you'll be taking a step towards achieving your target weight? The choice is yours!

The first time you do this will require the most effort, but on subsequent occasions it will gradually get easier. Eventually, you'll get to the point where the thought might still cross your mind that you like the look of that food, but your new way of dealing with it will be to think, *I'm not hungry, so I'm not going to eat it.*

You can hit your Pause Button whenever you need to give yourself a few seconds to take time out and think through a situation, reminding yourself of the possible consequences rather than just carrying on regardless and only facing the fallout after the event.

We recommend that people who want to use PBT do one of the following: obtain a PBT device or card, or one of our wristbands, from our website, www.pausebuttontherapy.com, just visualize a remote control device, or use the technique of crooking their index finger and pressing with the thumb − a 'virtual' remote control!

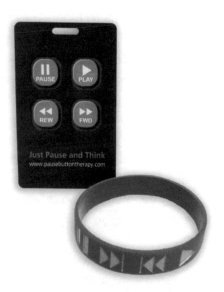

The PBT card and wristband

Incorporating PBT into Your Life

Here's the PBT sequence in six easy steps:

1. Identify the moment. That nanosecond when you need to press the Pause button and think 'stop'. This is the hardest part. It's learning which situations you need to stop and think about, and which you don't.

2. Press Pause. Now you're safe – nothing can 'get at you' and no one can influence you – your life has just been frozen for as long as you need it to be. This may just be a few seconds, or it may be longer.

3. Now use the Fast Forward Button to go forward to the future, whether it's an hour or a day ahead. See, smell, and feel the results of what you're about to do to get a clear, full-colour picture of the scene at the time. This allows you to experience in detail the ramifications of what you did – the effect that food you ate will have on your future, or the implications for your waistline of having those drinks – whatever it happens to be.

4. Now Rewind back to the present, and then Fast-Forward to the second option. Repeat the visualization process and see how much better you feel. Notice your new-found pride, and how positive, empowered, and in control you feel.

5. Once again, Rewind back to the present, and decide which of the actions you are going to take.

6. Press Play and get on with your life.

> *PBT can be summed up in four words:*
> *Pause, Think, Decide, Act*

Pause Button Therapy was introduced to a wider academic audience when we were privileged to be invited to make a presentation at the first ever International Conference on Time Perspective, in Portugal, in September 2012. We presented the results of a pilot experimental study aimed at examining PBT in relation to weight loss. Dr Theano Kalavana, of Cyprus University of Technology, wrote a paper explaining the role and level of success of PBT in the weight loss of a number of clients.

You can learn much more about how you can use PBT in your weight loss journey, and other aspects of your life, by reading our first book, *Pause Button Therapy*, published by Hay House.

Starting to Think Like a Slim Person

Some eating and drinking is habitual – it's 7 p.m. so you have a glass of wine. You're reacting to the thought that's set up the habit in the first place. On top of which, without a moment's thought, out comes a packet of crisps and, as if by magic, 200 unnecessary calories go around your waist, all in a heartbeat. A 'normal' eater would, with barely a thought, handle it differently. *I'll be eating in 10 minutes, so it'll spoil my appetite,* they think, or *I'm not stupid, or hungry – they're empty calories. I'll leave them for now, thank you very much!*

A slim person might snack, but they'll choose a banana, or five grapes, or a couple of green olives. How many peanuts or crisps would you have along with your glass of wine? Be honest. A slim person might have three or four, or – of course – none at all.

Once you've got into the habit of stopping yourself *before* you start to eat, to ask the question, you should find it easy to develop an automatic process. Not before every forkful, just at the beginning of every 'eating episode'. Then, as you go through the meal, you need to recognize the feeling that your hunger is subsiding and you're beginning to feel satisfied, and stop at that point.

Every time you eat to normal fullness, give yourself credit for it – tell yourself you're exercising and so strengthening your 'resistance muscle'. The opposite is equally true: give in to temptation more often and it's your 'giving-in muscle' that will get stronger.

> *You'll find that you latch on to some of these ideas more than others, but together they'll give you the clues as to how you can start thinking like a slim person. And you can.*

So, you're starting to redefine your levels of feeling full. That's one critical piece of the jigsaw. Some people have a big plateful at mealtimes, and never eat between meals. Others will eat normally, or maybe even not eat very much at all in front of other people, then work their way through a whole packet of biscuits when they're alone, permanently grazing between meals, yet making out in public that they don't really eat much.

There are different viewpoints to help you see the ways you can begin to change. NLP is often used in tandem with the hypnotherapy element of PBT – it's about learning to see yourself from a different perspective. An example of NLP is the 'going there first' that we explored earlier, i.e. if you're a size 18, or 20, close your eyes and imagine yourself on a date in the future, as a size 12.

Try to recognize in detail what you'll smell like and feel like; how much confidence you'll have; how much energy you'll have; the acknowledgement you'll be getting from others; where you'll be going that evening; what you'll be eating; what your friends will say to you; how happy you'll feel, etc.

Another example would be to look at the difference between yourself and someone who has the correct relationship with food and try to model yourself on that person. What does that person do with food that is different?

Or imagine yourself in a pair of jeans or a top that you haven't been able to wear for a while. If you *really* imagine yourself – see yourself in the jeans in your mind's eye, visualize how you will look walking into a party in that fashionable outfit – it's a positive image. It's all to do with feeling better about yourself. You'll see how you feel with improved self-esteem, a better self-image. Instead of all the negative feedback you've been pouring on yourself, you can project yourself into a better, slimmer future.

FOOD ISN'T A SECURITY BLANKET

When 40-year-old Mark M. bumped into a friend he hadn't seen in months and didn't recognize her because of her noticeable weight loss, he learned about the Gastric Mind Band. As a result, he made the choice to use the GMB system with Hazel Newsom in the USA. 'Hazel made me realize I'd been using food as a security blanket of sorts,' he says, 'not as fuel for my body.'

Having lost 70lb (32kg) when he spoke to us about his GMB journey, Mark said he felt better about 'everything!' 'I've gained a huge amount of confidence – life is just way better now that I've conquered that monkey on my back. I'm now hyper-aware of what I put in my body, and chalk my success up to that. Awareness, understanding, and self-confidence: those are the major factors.

'It was all pretty easy; I think I was just ready for it. My eating pattern is still different over a year later. It's become my new pattern. You don't have to give up all the foods you like; you just eat a healthier version and amount of it!'

Changing Your Filter

Staying on the subject of visualization, it's possible, even though it sounds a bit odd, to acknowledge your internal voices – the ones you've seen as critical. If you make friends with them, filter out criticism and listen to support and encouragement, it can help you achieve inner harmony.

Everyone tends to see things through their own 'filters', which are based on their experiences. For example, two women walking along a pavement see two men coming towards them, one of whom is wearing a baseball cap. One of the women had a bad experience as a kid when watching a film in which the baddie wore a baseball cap, so she's got this idea that anyone wearing a baseball cap is bad, and she starts having a panic attack. The other woman greets the men with a friendly 'hello'. The guy in the baseball cap is an off-duty policeman, and is the woman's cousin. So there are completely different filters for these two women, according to their past experiences.

Now is the time for you to start removing your filters, and boost the positive. If, when you look in the mirror, you continually criticize the way you look, saying negative things like, 'I'm frumpy', 'I can't wear nice clothes', or 'I'm ugly', you're putting your own filters on your image. You'll find that your other half loves you because of who you are; they don't see you as overweight and frumpy at all. It's all been down to your negative filter.

Now for Some Straight Talking

Do you accept responsibility for your situation, and the consequences of your actions? If you believe you do, you need to start thinking about why you're fat and why you've done nothing about it so far.

Would it destabilize you, mess with your head a bit, if we asked how you managed to get so large? How you manage to maintain your current weight? Do you think it's a weird question? You've probably not been asked it before. So, how *do* you manage? It must be hard work to stay a size 16, 18, 24, 32? It must take so much effort. Wouldn't it be better to put in a bit of effort to become slimmer and maintain *that* size?

What do you *really* want, what do you *dream* of? Can you see the end result if you close your eyes?

If you went to the beach and saw a sign saying 'Strong undercurrents, risk of drowning, do not swim in the water', you wouldn't go in the sea. But you'll go out and have a cheeseburger and chips. What's the difference between these actions? Is it that having that one cheeseburger and chips isn't going to kill you?

If we took you to a zebra crossing, put a blindfold on you and said, 'Go on, walk across that', you might get to the other side and say, 'Yeah, I've done it!' Then you'd want to cross it again because you managed it the first time. But, just because that one cheeseburger didn't kill you, it doesn't mean you can eat one as often as you like, because the chances are that one day one of them will.

Often, people will cherry-pick the advice they're willing to believe. You may have read, years ago, that an aspirin a day thins the blood, helping you to avoid stroke, or deep-vein thrombosis, or whatever. So you've taken an aspirin a day for the past nine years. But the same newspaper where you read about aspirin has been saying monthly, weekly, maybe even daily, that you should try to keep your BMI below 25. Did you follow that piece of advice? Or was it too much like hard work?

Why don't you try out a Zimmer frame for a while? You may have an elderly or disabled friend or relative you could borrow one from. Go on, give it a try. You may find it funny, but if you carry on with your poor eating habits, it'll be anything but funny. You may need to get used to it for real.

All feelings and emotions are constructive. Even if they're painful, they are there to tell us something, whether good or bad – but the correct action should be taken. When the temperature light flashes on the dashboard of your car, you don't fill up with fuel. When the petrol light comes on, no one pulls into a garage and tops up with oil. So why, when you're bored, would you even *consider* eating a packet of crisps? Wouldn't reading a book, going for a walk, or watching a movie be a more appropriate reaction?

Why do we do it?

If you're faced with choices and are struggling, just take a walk outside and do anything to slow the situation down. Go outside and think about it, press your Pause Button, and then go back in.

SARAH JAYNE HART'S STORY

In spring 2012, it's likely that a sizeable proportion of the UK population saw images of Sarah Jayne Hart – in newspapers, on TV and in magazines. Photographs of her were broadcast further afield, too – in Australia and the USA. One of our more visible success stories, Sarah's weight-loss journey is, in essence, the same as that of anyone going through GMB; she may have had more weight to lose than many, perhaps, but she had the same issues.

Although she would once have described herself as a 'typical bubbly fat girl', Sarah admits now that she was 'just dying inside'. She was 19 – and 19 stone (121kg) when she got married in a double wedding with her sister Amanda in 1990. And nine years down the line, it was the wedding photos of Sarah, alongside her petite size 8 sibling, that helped spur her on to shed the excess weight – with our help, of course.

Now fit and healthy, and weighing in at 9½–10 stone (60–63kg), the 5ft 4in (1.63m) travel agent from Caerphilly, Wales, had piled on weight as a girl due to unhealthy eating habits and steroid treatment for her asthma. At the age of 14 she was 14 stone (88.9kg). At the time, she maintained that her classmates' teasing didn't affect her, but admits now that she was putting on a 'bubbly' persona – the clichéd fat happy person.

By the time of her wedding to Lee, Sarah's denial was covering a larger weight problem. Her size 24 wedding dress had to be made specially for her. 'I was in love and happy,' she says, 'but looking back at the wedding photos, I was shocked. I never realized I was that big.'

Marriage saw Sarah enjoying calorie-laden evening meals such as curry and pasta dishes. She also enjoyed snacking on crisps, pies and pasties. After the birth of her two sons, Harrison and Marshall, Sarah's weight kept rising, peaking at 21 stone (133.kg). Her BMI was 50, which classified her as 'super morbidly obese'.

Time to Make a Change

In summer 2008 she'd attempted to slim down, but only dropped about 12lb (5.5kg) until that Christmas, flying home to the UK from France where she and Lee were living, she suffered the classic indignity of being unable to do up the seat belt. At a New Year's Eve party she went as an angel but felt 'absolutely disgusting'. 'I looked awful – it was just like a big white tent,' she says. 'I looked at those pictures and thought, *I've got to sort myself out.*'

Sarah made a New Year's resolution and no one but she knew how determined she was to see it through. 'I'd seen an article about a girl who'd lost lots of weight with GMB, and I thought it was the answer to all my prayers. I couldn't afford to pay for a gastric band, and anyway it's a big step. I thought if I could just reprogramme how I think…'

So how quickly did GMB take effect? 'I started losing weight immediately,' she recalls. 'I began by eating the kind of food that you eat after gastric band surgery – like soup – but then I tried to cut out carbs as much as possible. They'd been my biggest downfall – I used to love pasta, bread and butter – but I can't eat them now. I know I'll feel 10 times worse, and there's no point. I'd rather eat a healthy salad and enjoy that, and I'm not beating myself up about it!'

She has more of a sweet tooth today. 'Now I'll have a couple of sweets or something, but that'll satisfy me. Once I'd eat a McDonald's and it wouldn't fill me, or an

Indian meal – that was my favourite – but I haven't had one since starting GMB.

'For breakfast now I either have cereal or yoghurt, or a cereal bar. Lunch is usually a salad or soup; in the afternoon I'll have another yoghurt/cereal bar and then meat and salad for dinner. Food doesn't bother me now – I can walk into the local sandwich bar and buy lunch for myself and others, or go into a Burger King at the airport. These places aren't a worry for me any more. It's just choosing. I get the odd day when I want something, but it's very rare. I don't have it, though. At McDonald's now I'll have the healthiest thing on the menu. I just don't fancy the burger.

'I never believed I could think like this, but GMB has totally changed my mindset. Even on holiday I won't let myself slip at all. If I go to a restaurant I'll choose a chicken salad or something and I'm more than happy with that. Even a salad is a treat, because with dressing it could be a bit naughty!

Going Beyond Target

Now a steady size 8–10, with a normal BMI of 22–24, Sarah still has vivid memories of what being fat felt like. 'I can tell now that people are fattist. You don't realize it at the time, but people look at you in a different way. Strangers are friendlier towards me now. And before, when I'd walk through a car park, I'd wonder whether I could fit between two parked cars. Then there's my kids. By being overweight, I was putting myself at so much more risk of health problems, and I didn't want to be the fat mum at school – not after my nephew got teased when I took him once.'

Sarah initially hoped to lose a couple of stone. 'I definitely didn't expect the results I got,' she says. 'I'd always said I wanted to get to 14 stone (89kg). My illusion was that I was going to be happy to be a size 14/16; I didn't want to be thin. Then, when I got to that weight, I didn't want to stay there, so I set myself another goal of 12 stone (76kg) – and when I got there I felt the same again and set my goal at being under 10 stone (63kg) and that's where I am now.

'I was very focused – I wanted it to work and that's why it was successful. I just thought, it's all in the mind, and it literally reprogrammed how I think of food and my relationship with food. It was almost like it changed my thoughts.

'I was surprised how much therapy was involved with GMB – talking about my relationship with food and opening up about it. I didn't realize some of the issues I had; for example, I didn't realize how greedy I was until I talked about it. Compared with what I eat now, I'm shocked by how much greed I had in me.

'I'm so afraid of slipping but I know that I won't,' Sarah says. 'I'm happy with the way I look, but there's always that little moment… maybe a bloated belly. When I was large I could never understand how someone slim thought like that, but now I realize that you can just tell – how your clothes feel for example. I'm getting to the point where I'll buy clothes in sizes 8–10. I've gone through stages of buying a bigger size, thinking a small size wouldn't fit me. I've got to learn to live with myself. I did keep my big clothes for a while, but that's only like saying to yourself that you'll need them.'

A Brand New Lifestyle

'My biggest motivation wasn't wanting to glam up to go out – I always tried my best at that. It was to look nice in casual clothes, day to day. To go to the pub in jeans and a T-shirt – I looked awful in jeans before. When I go out with my friends now, instead of having to put up with some drunk person making comments about the size of my arms, it's lovely. I can share clothes with my friends and my sister, too, and be more involved in things. It's true that I did fall out with my sister for a while, after she told me some home truths. We had a turbulent relationship, but we always get over things like that.'

Sarah's now an exercise fiend, and has run a half-marathon, with another planned. 'I love being active; I just couldn't do it before. I would try to go to the gym but I wasn't motivated because the fitness and the healthy eating go together. I can't understand how people can't do both. I wouldn't have lost half the weight without exercising. I have found that it's really good for the mind, too.

'It shocks me how fit I am now – at the boot camp I was the third fittest out of about 15 of us. Before, I would have been struggling to do all the activities. When I was fat, things were difficult for me. I couldn't even do the housework without feeling exhausted.

'In the past, I tried everything under the sun – all the diets, pills, everything. Everybody talks about diet food and slimming food, and asks me if I'm allowed to eat this, or that. That's where I can see that my relationship with food is different. I can eat whatever I want – I can choose. And I don't want to eat junk. It's just choosing.

'I'd say the therapy is really good. There's a lot of hard work, and you've got to put it in yourself, but I think GMB just reprogrammes your mind to rethink your relationship with food. It's brilliant. I don't feel like I'm on a diet. I can eat whatever I choose – it's just making the right choices.'

WHAT YOU'VE LEARNED IN THIS CHAPTER
. . . .

- There are meals that matter and meals that don't.
- You have to retrain your subconscious mind over a period of time.
- Everything starts with a thought.
- To watch out for the Diet Terrorists.
- How to use your Pause Button.

Chapter 12
Session 4: The Gastric Mind Band

This session is the one in which the Gastric Mind Band itself is implanted into the subconscious mind using self-hypnosis.

Before getting to this stage, you should have developed a clear idea of how you became overweight in the first place; why you want to become a healthier weight, and the tools you're going to use to achieve this. The imagery of 'implanting' a Gastric Mind Band is there to back the whole process up – to give you another, final, tool in your toolbox.

This is the last session, so, a bit like with a surgical gastric band, the process is reaching the point where it becomes 'all up to you'. Some of what you're about to read has been explored earlier in the book, but it does no harm to repeat things if it helps you to learn how to change your flawed relationship with food.

Reading this chapter will add the finishing touch to your journey towards shedding your excess weight. You'll have your own way of imagining a tightening, or shrinking, of your stomach. As you read on, keep reminding yourself of the size of the smaller 'pouch-sized' capacity you are aiming to achieve for your stomach.

Think of a golf ball. Get hold of a real one if you can, and keep it in your hand as you read this chapter.

Revisiting the Surgical Gastric Band

Before we continue, though, let's take another look at the surgical gastric band.

A typical adult stomach is about 30.5cm (12in) long, and is 15.2cm (6in) across at its widest point; it holds around 1.14 litres (2 pints).[1] The whole purpose of the gastric band is to restrict the amount of food a person can physically eat at one sitting. It does this by reducing the capacity of their stomach.

The band works on the same principle as a cable tie, with a one-way locking catch. It's wrapped around the outside of the top part of the stomach and clicked into place, and, because the stomach is soft, the band nips it in, changing the shape and creating a small pouch in the stomach's upper section. This pouch is literally about the size of a golf ball.

Once the gastric band is fitted, whatever food is eaten simply gathers in the pouch, and as soon as this is full, the person experiences the feeling of fullness (though higher up in the abdomen than usual) and cannot physically cram any more food in. The size of a meal that someone with a gastric band can eat is only equal to 5–6 tablespoons (75–90ml) of food. Compare this to a meal size of around two clenched fists, which is what it would take to fill a normal stomach.

Then, very slowly, the food 'drip feeds' through the narrow opening at the bottom of the stomach pouch, and passes into the lower part of the stomach, where the digestive enzymes in the stomach acid break it all down, so it can then pass through the intestines in the normal way.[2] So, basically, the person feels full after eating just a very small amount of food, and then they will stay feeling satisfied for a long time afterwards, because it takes so long for all the food to filter down through the narrow gap.

If you imagine eating such a small amount of food without having the band in place, firstly you wouldn't actually feel very satisfied. Also, you would start to feel hungry again in a short time, because the food would be able to pass relatively quickly through the stomach and into the intestines. The band simply slows down the whole process and allows the person to feel very satisfied after a tiny amount of food. Just as it's designed to do.

An overweight person will be used to eating larger than necessary portions of food, and their stomach will be stretched – anyone's stomach can distend by as much as 50 times its empty volume,[3] and the overweight person will have created a larger 'memory' of fullness in their stomach and possibly even stretched it,[4] which of course means they have a big hole to fill every time they eat!

Then, after the surgery, things change drastically. From eating vast quantities before the operation, the person then has to get used to tiny portion sizes. On top of that, they have to take mouthfuls no bigger than the size of the rubber on the end of a pencil, or roughly the size of the nail on their little finger.

Each mouthful then has to be chewed at least 10 times before it can be swallowed, otherwise the food particles will be too big to pass through the pouch opening and the food will sit there, causing a blockage until it ends up making a sudden reappearance as the body rejects it! There's even a special name for this phenomenon – it's called 'productive burping'. How nice!

Having a gastric band fitted does not teach you how to eat normally. What is going on in your head controls everything, and if your head isn't sorted out properly, you will find ways to cheat the band.

So, the actual surgery is all pretty drastic, really. What a difference – going from gulping down massive portions of food – shovelling it in as fast as possible, chewing a couple of times and it's gone – to suddenly taking forever to eat tiny amounts of food in mousetrap-sized pieces and chewing it to death!

GASTRIC BAND SURGERY: IS IT WORTH THE RISK?

Gastric band surgery carries a risk of death – around 1 in 1,000–2,000 people will die as a result of having the operation.[5] Now, if you imagine that someone was selling you a lottery ticket with a one in 2,000 chance of winning, you'd want to buy quite a few, wouldn't you? After all, those odds are pretty good. When it's your life you're talking about, though, maybe you should be thinking: 'Hang on a minute, I don't know if I want to take that risk.'

After gastric band surgery, you have to change your eating habits in more ways than one. At your 4–5 meals a day, you're advised to eat your food in a certain order. For example, choosing the meat first, because you have to chew it thoroughly, which takes time – and also the meat will stay in the pouch for a long time.

Vegetables are the next in line, as they'll sit on top of the meat in the pouch; soft, mushy things like mashed potato have to be saved until last. If you ate the meal in reverse order, the food would pass through the pouch easily and you'd be able to eat more, which, of course, defeats the whole object of having the band fitted in the first place!

It's only healthy, solid food that needs chewing which gets restricted by the gastric band. Things that can easily be reduced to a liquid consistency – chocolate, ice cream, typical comfort foods – will actually pass through the band very easily.

If a comfort eater who makes the wrong food choices and eats meals at the wrong time has the operation, they'll come to after the operation and nothing will have changed. They are still going to be a comfort eater; they're still going to eat the wrong food at the wrong times, and make the wrong choices. The band won't actually stop them from doing these things. They still have to make the effort to be aware of what they're eating and why.

It's not unheard of for people to be told they actually need to put weight on in order to qualify for the gastric band operation!

Not a Miracle Cure

The gastric band operation is not foolproof, and its success is not 100 per cent guaranteed. A lot of people don't seem to realize this. They think that it's a magic wand, guaranteed to solve everything, and that they're not going to have to make any changes or put in any effort because the band will do it all for them. The reality is very different. A surgical band only has a success rate of around 66 per cent in the longer term.[6]

And about a third of people who have the operation will get around the band and cheat on it. In order to satisfy their 'need' for junk food, some people put everything – burgers, fries, milkshakes, you name it – in a blender and then drink the resulting puree. It just goes to prove how powerful the human mind is. If your head is not in the right place, it can just sabotage what you want to do.

You're also advised not to eat and drink at the same time.[7] Not drinking for anything up to an hour before and after a meal is a rule which varies from provider to provider; the reasons also vary, but here are a few of them:

- Liquids can help to flush food through the pouch faster, thereby making it possible to eat again sooner.

- Liquids taken after food can 'settle' on top of the pouch, making its contents heavier and increasing the likelihood of stretching and band slippage.

- Some patients experience vomiting if they drink during a meal.

Obviously none of this applies with GMB. We want eating to be an enjoyable experience, and for it to be perfectly normal to sit and have a meal and a drink at the same time. As we've said before, the operation doesn't change the thinking of a comfort eater, or the way in which they make their choices.

In the end, if you just change your approach to food, you shouldn't need to have a surgical gastric band for the rest of your life. People tend to rely on the band to do everything for them, rather than relying on their own mind, so they often expect to have the band for life. And, of course, if they're not successful and don't lose weight, then it's very easy to blame it all on the band, rather than accept responsibility for their failure.

Having the operation doesn't actually help people to build a normal, healthy relationship with food; it's just like being on a diet in which you end up being even more obsessed with food.

Not only that, but the food you'll find harder to eat with the surgical band is the healthy kind... there's no such difficulty with junk food.

The Final GMB Tool

Okay, at this point our clients, and you the reader, have all the tools in your GMB toolbox. All but one: the Gastric Mind Band.

Clench your fist. That's about the size of your stomach (or at least it would be if you hadn't stretched it through overeating!). Look at it again. Not very big, is it? How on earth do you fit all that food in there when you overeat? Well, the next step is to picture your stomach shrinking. Hold that golf ball in your dominant hand. Hold it and squeeze. Shut your eyes and feel the size of it. Now that's really not very big at all, is it? But it's the size of the pouch created by a surgical gastric band, and it's what you'll be visualizing as your capacity for food. Squeeze it again.

In the clinic, clients go through the entire process of mentally having a gastric band fitted under hypnotherapy. They are 'taken' down hospital corridors, hear reassuring voices, and receive all the imagery to suggest that they've had sedation and an anaesthetic in a hospital... all under hypnosis.

If you are still reading the book, your motivation has carried you this far. If you want to shed your excess weight enough, by now you'll be working hard to retrain your conscious mind. And through self-hypnosis, visualizing the golf ball should be enough of an image to convince your subconscious that your stomach has a smaller capacity now.

Wearing a GMB wristband is a helpful memory-jogger, signifying the control the Gastric Mind Band will have on the everyday eating choices of those who've undergone the process in one of our clinics. It's a tangible reminder of the changes taking place in the mind and the stomach. For details of availability of the bands, visit www.gmband.com

If you'd had gastric band surgery, your next few weeks would involve consuming soup, blended or liquidized food… nothing to get your teeth into. Without surgery there's obviously no actual band, so there's no need for this, but don't be surprised, if, like some clinic clients, you experience a significant reduction in how much you feel able to eat following your experience of the Gastric Mind Band procedure, as the mind is a very powerful tool.

Take it gently to begin with; start with very small portions of healthy nutritious food – which you'll almost certainly have been doing since the first session anyway, because you will have been questioning all your food choices.

But if there are times when you really do want a piece of chocolate, just allow yourself to have it, because this whole process is not about having forbidden foods. When you set up the idea that something is 'forbidden', it's typical to want it more. Deprivation creates a stronger desire.

You can eat whatever you want to eat, but always consider first whether what you choose to eat is going to help you or hinder you. And, above all, make sure you are definitely hungry before you eat anything – it doesn't matter whether it's chocolate or a carrot – if you're not hungry you *don't* need it!

Did we really say you can have a piece of chocolate? Well, yes, we certainly did. GMB is about eating in the real world, enjoying your food and your life but not letting your food take over your life. You have the control. Eat moderately most of the time and you'll give yourself options.

Everything you're doing now, all your actions, are supposed to be helping you achieve this ultimate goal – this thing that is the most important in your life: the reason why you've picked up and read this book.

Your Gastric Mind Band self-hypnosis is coming up, but first you might like to think about what happens once the initial GMB process is complete:

A Few Weeks Later...

In the same way as if you'd had a surgical gastric band fitted, we suggest you have a 'post-treatment' session to assess how you're progressing, and if necessary, adjust the 'grip' that the band – in your case the Mind Band – has on your eating habits.

You'll probably have been checking your weight/ measurements weekly, or possibly more often. Beware weighing yourself too often, though, because that can give a misleading view of what's happening in the bigger picture. Four to six weeks after you started this process is a good time to sit back and assess how much you've changed your thinking, and how much this altered thinking has changed your eating.

These new eating habits should, in turn, have had an effect on the scales; if it's not quite as fast as you'd like, you could revisit the earlier sessions and see what hit home for you the most; see whether there's a way to 'tweak' your thinking still further.

What you should avoid is 'expecting miracles yesterday'. We've said it before but it could do with repeating – the Gastric Mind Band is a life change. It's not a diet, or a quick cure, but rather a weight management system that *you design for your own way of living,* because everyone's different.

Just to help you remember: how long did it take you to put the weight on? Getting rid of the excess weight won't be an overnight thing!

There's no point at all in doing this for a few weeks and then letting go and reverting to your old ways – although if you've read carefully from start to finish, and really got the picture from answering the questionnaire, you'll have had the best chance of putting into practice our techniques for avoiding overeating from that point on.

If you're starting to doubt yourself and how much you've really changed, shut your eyes and take yourself back to the fork in the road. A year ahead, being exactly the same as you are now, or maybe even heavier, or a year ahead having lost weight consistently and feeling good about yourself. Which makes you feel better? There's no question! Besides, if you've shed *any* of that excess weight, you should be in a better place mentally than you were a few weeks back, don't you think?

As you approach your target weight, you should allow yourself another period of time – maybe an hour, maybe a day, whatever you need – for reflecting on how your eating habits and your choices have changed, and the difference it's made to your life. There's every chance you'll have altered all the patterns of your attitude to food in such a way that you don't really need to think about it. You're already there.

It's not necessarily at target – but then target is what you make it. Certainly you're a different eater, and probably a different shopper. Maybe even a different person. But you're the person you've always known you could be, yet until now hadn't found the *motivation* to be.

At Your Target Weight and Beyond

Once you reach your target weight, we suggest a final session of self-hypnosis to 'release' the grip of the Gastric Mind Band in the same way that surgical gastric band patients would have some saline removed from the band, enabling them to start eating the right amount of food to maintain their weight rather than to continue to reduce it.

You, having read this book and started on your journey to shed your excess weight, will be taking sole responsibility for your own follow-up! If you're shedding, or have finished shedding, your excess weight, you need only reread the book (or those bits which caught your imagination most powerfully) from time to time.

Allow yourself a self-hypnosis session every so often, choosing as your Positive Thoughts those elements of your journey that mean the most to you. Whether it's something you feel particularly proud to have achieved, or something you're aware is a weak point, it's up to you. But every time you reinforce what you've learned, your subconscious will be a stronger ally in your journey to be and remain a healthy weight.

WHAT YOU'VE LEARNED IN THIS CHAPTER
. . . .

- Your subconscious mind should begin to help you notice a restriction in your stomach capacity.

- Eating smaller quantities of food will come naturally.

- To maintain your weight loss, you must read, reread and keep rereading this book. You know it makes sense!

Chapter 13
Self-Hypnosis 3

In the first self-hypnosis session we explained how, with the motivation for change, you can provide a boost to your subconscious mind by relaxing yourself deeply. If you want to remind yourself of the process, you will find it on page 119.

Please note that self-hypnosis should never be practised when driving, operating machinery or carrying out any other activity that requires your full attention.

For this session it will help if you can have a golf ball with you.

Choose at least three relevant and appropriate Positive Thoughts from the list on page 237, and read and revise them. You need to be able to repeat them to yourself mentally at least three times. They are your messages to your subconscious mind to change your behaviour for life, starting now.

If there are more than three appropriate Positive Thoughts, you can alternate and choose a different set each time you do this session.

Read your Positive Thoughts and make sure you feel completely focused on what you are trying to achieve before you set about relaxing, so you don't have to 'wake up' to refer to notes, or remind yourself what you meant to concentrate on. It's the subconscious mind you want to target, and that is best addressed when you are deeply relaxed.

You now need to 'talk' yourself into a state of deep relaxation.

- You should fix your gaze on a point, so choose something to concentrate on. Then say three or four times, 'I am going to count down from five to one; my eyelids are getting heavy and at one I will close my eyes and be completely relaxed.'

- Now, slowly and silently, count down from five to one, taking a deep breath between each number. When you reach one, close your eyes, and with another, deeper, breath, release and relax.

- Now concentrate on every part of your body as a rolling sequence, starting with your feet or your head. Release the tension from each part, and relax your muscles as you go. Repeat silently something like, 'Let go, release, relax'.

- Now picture an evocative set of steps — 10 of them — leading down to somewhere you know you'll be safe and at ease. You can choose — countryside, beach, a snowy mountain — it's up to you and your imagination and what makes you feel comfortable.

- Count down from 10 to 1, and at one you should see yourself in that secluded, special place, all alone. Take time to settle down; get used to what's around you — the sounds, the smells, the breeze, tastes... The more you can visualize, the more focused and successful the session will be.

You should now imagine yourself at the start of a brand new life. You're so carried away with all those wonderful, positive feelings that you hardly notice yourself pick up the golf ball in your dominant hand. Squeeze that golf ball in your hand, really focusing your attention on the size and dimensions of your stomach, which is much, much smaller – the size of that ball. Squeeze again and become aware of a tightening feeling in your stomach now. In your mind's eye, picture a band being wrapped around the top of your stomach. The tightening feeling is much stronger now, and you can picture how your stomach has been reduced in size.

For the final session, your Positive Thoughts are as follows:

1. You know that your brand new life starts now.

2. You're on your journey to becoming permanently slimmer and healthier.

3. Your excess weight, which you're going to get rid of, has been weighing you down and holding you back from being the person you really want to be.

4. Your lifestyle will now include smaller portions of food, and total control of your weight and size.

5. Thinking about this is relaxing and not at all stressful – you are confident, positive, and full of excitement about how your life is changing for the better.

6. The golf ball in your hand is going to help you identify just how much smaller your stomach capacity is going to be.

7. You are now more aware of your stomach – as if you were having gastric band surgery – and squeezing the golf ball

helps you focus your attention on the size of your stomach in the past and now.

8. You can picture how your stomach has been reduced in size.

9. The more you squeeze the ball, the tighter your stomach feels.

10. You will find that just a small amount of food is all you want and need to eat at each meal, though you feel totally satisfied.

11. If you try to eat more food than you need, your stomach will feel very uncomfortable. If you stop eating, you'll feel more comfortable and completely satisfied.

12. Food is no longer a comfort or an emotional crutch – it's a source of nourishment and nothing more.

13. You can adjust your 'golf ball' whenever you choose, shedding your excess weight at a rate to suit you.

14. This is a permanent way of life.

You're now ready to start your new, healthy life.

Now count yourself up from one to five, suggesting that you have enjoyed a wonderful relaxation, and on five you will open your eyes, feeling refreshed and energized.

If you decide to do your self-hypnosis before going to sleep, you can suggest that on the count of five, you will move into a normal and natural sleep until it's time for you to wake.

PART 3
MOVING FORWARD

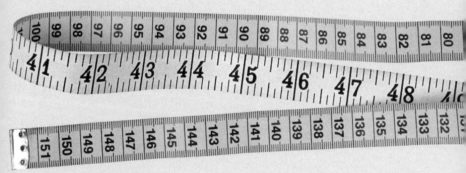

Chapter 14
A Reminder of the Health Risks of Obesity

It's definitely worth labouring the point that our list of obesity-related illnesses earlier in the book wasn't exhaustive. Even what you're about to read is not the full story: just do some research for yourself. In the meantime, here's some more to think about.

Type 2 Diabetes

This is reckoned to be the fourth or fifth largest killer in most developed countries. More than three quarters of people with Type 2 diabetes are overweight. Statistically, overweight people are twice as likely to develop Type 2 diabetes as those of normal weight. Research has indicated that in the Western world more than 90 per cent of cases of Type 2 diabetes are attributable to weight gain.

Women who have a BMI greater than 35.0 are more than 93 times more at risk of developing the disease than women with a normal BMI. The connection between obesity and diabetes is as strong as that between smoking and lung cancer, but it just doesn't seem to get the media attention.

The complications of Type 2 diabetes can lead to loss of sight, kidney problems and more. In more severe cases, sufferers have to keep a very close watch on what they eat and drink, test their blood or urine daily or several times a day, and maybe inject themselves with insulin. The charity Diabetes UK says that research shows that losing weight can reduce the risk of developing Type 2 diabetes by 58 per cent.

Type 2 diabetes is often referred to as 'adult onset diabetes', as it was once rare for it to develop in childhood. However, in recent years, an increase in the number of overweight and obese children has resulted in an alarming rise in premature Type 2 diabetes.

Being overweight makes a person resistant to the hormone insulin, which carries sugar from the blood to the cells, where it's used for energy. When they become insulin resistant, the sugar can't pass into the cells and so it stays in their blood, making the blood sugar levels higher than normal.

This puts an extra strain on the cells that make insulin, as they try to bring the blood sugar levels back to normal, and eventually these cells could fail. Prolonged exposure to high blood glucose increases the risk of heart disease, stroke, high blood pressure, nerve damage, blindness, kidney failure, and poor circulation in the extremities, which can lead to amputation.[1]

Gallbladder Problems/Gallstones

Overweight people are seven times more likely to have gallstones than people who are of normal weight. Women are twice as likely develop gallstones as men, and also at risk are those who've recently followed an unhealthy weight-loss regime. Over 80 per cent of gallstones cases develop when the liver produces high-cholesterol-content bile – possibly due to a high cholesterol diet or an excess of refined carbohydrates like those found in white bread and cakes.

In women, the risk of developing gallstones or having the gallbladder removed completely (cholecystectomy) is about 20 per 1,000 women per year for those with a BMI greater than 40, compared with three per 1,000 in normal-weight women. Also, unlike other weight-related conditions, weight reduction in the morbidly obese patient actually *increases* the risk of gallstone formation, especially if the weight loss is rapid.[2]

Osteoarthritis

This is the most common cause of pain in older people, and the knees are the area most affected. When we walk, every step exerts a force on our knees of 1.5 times our whole body weight, and when we run, this force is increased to up to six times our body weight. The force exerted on the hips is estimated to be around three times our body weight.

Carrying extra weight puts a lot of pressure on all the joints, especially the knees. The extra pressure eventually wears away the cartilage, which normally forms a cushion between the bones, so the bones then grind together, making movement difficult and painful. Being just 10lb (4.5kg) overweight increases the force on the knee by 30–60lb (13.5–27kg) with each step we take.

Research has shown that obese women are four times more likely to develop arthritis in the knee joint compared with women who are of normal weight. For obese men, the risk is nearly five times greater. Even just a small amount of weight loss reduces the risk of developing osteoarthritis of the knee, and can also help to reduce the pain experienced by people who already have it.

Joint replacement operations on obese patients have a higher rate of complications than those on people who are of normal weight. Obese patients spend more time on the operating table, they need to stay in hospital for longer to recover after the operation, and they often require more nursing/rehabilitation during their prolonged recovery period.[3]

One UK health authority has decided not to refer obese patients with arthritis for NHS hip or knee replacements 'to ensure that taxpayers' money is used for maximum clinical effect', because anaesthesia for the obese patient is more difficult and they do less well after the operation.[4]

'The doctor of the future will give no medication, but will interest his patients in the care of the human frame, diet and in the cause and prevention of disease.'
THOMAS EDISON

Coronary Heart Disease and Stroke

These conditions are the leading causes of death and disability for both men and women in the Western world. Overweight people are more likely to have high blood pressure, and are three times more likely to be at risk from heart disease and stroke, than people who are not overweight. Very high blood levels of cholesterol and triglycerides (blood fats) can also lead to heart disease and are often linked to obesity.

Obesity also contributes to angina (chest pain caused by decreased oxygen to the heart) and sudden death from heart disease or stroke without any signs or symptoms. Reducing your weight by just 10 per cent can decrease your risk of developing heart disease.

Obesity and poor diet are high risk factors for stroke, which, according to the NHS, is the third largest killer in the UK. Conditions such as diabetes and high blood pressure, both of which are also linked with overweight, can cause strokes, too.[5] The gradual accumulation of plaque in the arteries in coronary heart disease can cause angina or a heart attack.[6]

TOO YOUNG TO HAVE A STROKE?

As you know, the risk of heart disease and stroke is dramatically increased in overweight people, and neither condition affects only the elderly. We once had a client at the clinic who wanted help with depression. He told us it was caused by the pressure he was under having to look after his 43-year-old wife following her stroke, which resulted in her losing virtually all use of her left arm and leg. It was almost impossible for her to visit the bathroom and clean herself without help. He said she had been overweight prior to the stroke.

Gout

Gout is a joint disease caused by high levels of uric acid in the blood. Uric acid sometimes forms into solid stone or crystal masses that become deposited in the joints. Gout is more common in overweight people than people of normal weight, and the risk of developing the disorder increases in parallel with an increase in weight.[7]

Back Problems

People who are overweight are more likely to have, or to have worse, back problems. In the UK, one in six working days lost is due to back pain, and osteoporosis, osteoarthritis, rheumatoid arthritis and lower back pain are all exacerbated by the extra strain that obesity exerts on the spine.[8]

Cancer

Cancer Research UK says major studies have confirmed that obesity increases the risk of developing various cancers, and the World Health Organization (WHO) says obesity is the most important known avoidable cause of cancer after tobacco. Some 13,000 people a year in the UK could avoid getting cancer if they maintained a healthy weight.[9]

The UK's NHS says that, combined with a lack of exercise, obesity contributes to one third of cancers of the colon, breast, kidney and stomach. In women, cancers associated with obesity are cancer of the uterus, gallbladder, cervix, ovary, breast, and colon. Overweight men are at greater risk of developing cancer of the colon, rectum, and prostate.[10]

Some researchers are looking into whether the immune system – the body's first defence against disease, including cancer – struggles to such an extent under the sheer volume of products taken into the body in an overweight person's unhealthy diet that it's unable to provide that defence efficiently.[11]

Colon Cancer

Research has revealed that people who are obese are two to three times more likely to develop colon cancer than those who are normal weight. In the USA, the five-year survival rate from colon cancer is 63 per cent, but in Europe it is just 43 per cent, possibly due to differing colon screening programmes.[12]

Breast Cancer

According to Cancer Research UK, scientists estimate that some 7–15 per cent of cases of breast cancer in the developed world are linked to obesity. Although obesity doesn't increase the risk of breast cancer before menopause, obese women have a 30 per cent higher risk of post-menopausal breast cancer. If the average lifetime risk of breast cancer is 1 in 9, an obese woman's risk is 1 in 7.

The charity says that young women also need to be aware of the risks of obesity. After the age of 18, putting on about 4 stone (25kg) increases the risk of breast cancer by 45 per cent and putting on 7st 12lb (50kg) doubles the risk. Recent studies show that obesity not only increases the risk of getting breast cancer, but also shortens the time until the return of the disease, and lowers survival rates.

Cancer of the Oesophagus (gullet)

Being overweight doubles the risk of developing this type of cancer; being obese can triple it. According to Cancer Research UK, it is estimated that about 37 per cent of oesophageal cancer cases are linked to obesity.

Cancer of the Uterus

Cancer Research UK says that more than a third of womb cancer cases in the UK are linked to being overweight or obese.

Other Types of Cancer

Cancer Research UK says there is evidence of increased risk of the following types of cancer in people who are overweight or obese: cancer of the thyroid, ovary, pancreas, kidney, gallbladder, brain and liver; leukaemia; multiple myeloma (cancer of plasma cells in bone marrow); non-Hodgkin lymphoma; and aggressive prostate cancer.[13]

Asthma

A Harvard Medical School research study, published in the US *Archives of Internal Medicine* in November 1999, showed that the risk of developing asthma grew with increasing BMI, and so obese people can be almost three times more likely to develop it than non-obese people. The study, led by Dr Carlos A. Camargo Jr, involved 85,911 female registered nurses.[14]

> *When diet is wrong, medicine is of no use.*
> *When diet is correct, medicine is of no need.*
> **ANCIENT AYURVEDIC PROVERB**

Sleep Apnoea

Sleep apnoea – short periods (usually no more than a few seconds) without breathing during sleep followed by rousing when breathing restarts – may seem a relatively minor side effect of obesity, but for people who suffer from it, stopping breathing up to 300–500 times a night has a major impact on their performance during waking hours.

Obesity is the main risk factor for sleep apnoea, with neck diameters of over 43cm (17in) being the critical dimension. Not only are sufferers depleted of vital oxygen, but their night-time rest is so disturbed that they can have severe problems of sleepiness during the day – whether at work, driving, or whatever they are doing.[15]

Non-Alcoholic Fatty Liver Disease

Obesity is a risk factor in this disease, which includes in its spectrum fibrosis (scarring) and in the worst cases, cirrhosis and liver failure.[16]

> *'Let nothing which can be treated*
> *by diet be treated by other means.'*
> **MAIMONIDES**

Depression

How often have you heard (or said) the cliché about overweight people being 'fat but happy'? The statistics, however, suggest that the reality is very different. According to research published in the *Archives of General Psychiatry*, there are links between obesity and depression.[17] Researchers found that obese people have a 55 per cent increased risk of developing depression over time, and in fact, it works both ways: depressed people are at 58 per cent increased risk of becoming obese.

Infertility

The effects of obesity on the hormones of women of childbearing age can lead to irregular cycles, an increased risk of miscarriage and less success in IVF treatment.[18] Overweight or obese men are also more likely to have a low sperm count or fewer viable sperm.[19]

ARE YOU AN APPLE OR A PEAR?

When fat is concentrated around the abdomen and in the upper part of the body (the 'apple' shape), this poses a higher health risk than fat that settles around the hips (the 'pear' shape). Fat cells in the upper part of the body appear to have different qualities from those found in the lower parts. In fact, studies suggest a higher risk for diabetes in apple-shaped people and a lower risk in those who are pear-shaped.[20]

HOW BIG IS YOUR WAIST?

Another factor in determining the health risks of your body shape is the ratio of your waist size to that of your hips. Your waist-to-hip ratio (divide the size of your waist by that of your hips) should ideally be no greater than 0.8 for women and 0.9 for men.

Chapter 15
Your GMB Journey Continues

If you've read this far into the book, you should have already started your own weight loss and healthy eating process. Maybe you've already lost a little weight: if so, well done! Enjoy! But, here's the rub – you've possibly been here before, having lost weight. This time though, the sinking feeling that you're on the verge of putting it all back on within the next few weeks or months will not affect you. Because you know you've changed, right?

You've taken all those long hard looks at yourself and your previous bad eating habits, and you've got our words ringing in your ears about not eating unless you are hungry, not being a prisoner if you go out to dinner, not fooling yourself about how much you need to eat, remembering that a lapse isn't a disaster, and so on, so this time you've got all the tools you need each and every time you make food choices. Whether it's in the supermarket or your own kitchen, a 3-star Michelin restaurant or a friend's dinner party, you need never make the same mistakes again.

You've also learned how to relax yourself so deeply that you can revisit all your Positive Thoughts any time you choose, knowing they'll keep you on that high road to success.

So, if you're now expecting a chapter about what to do to maintain your new weight, that was it. Just keep doing what you've been doing. Eat mindfully, enjoy your food because you're eating *because you're hungry*, and above all, be happy! The toolkit worked!

GMB for Successful Dieters

Of course, you may be one of the many people who manage to shed excess weight easily enough on your own but find the problems start just as you should be beginning your new, happier, slimmer and healthier life. What problems? Keeping that weight off, we hear you say. And why? Because you revert to your old – bad – eating habits. It's as simple as that.

After your weight loss you might not even have returned to your bad relationship with food – perhaps you've just shed that weight for the first time and heard so much about the vicious circle of yo-yo dieting that you want to avoid it at all costs. Then again, you could be one of those unfortunate yo-yo dieters whose lives have been caught up in a repeated battle to shed weight, seemingly incapable of keeping it off.

How GMB can help is pretty straightforward. You've done what many would see as the hard bit, and now you're all set to feel and be positive. Having read the book and, at the same time begun to enjoy your life as the new, slimmer you, you've started to learn how and why you got fat in the first place and how to change your approach to food.

Rereading this book, and redoing the self-hypnosis sessions, is probably the best way to be sure of not slipping back and undoing all the good work you've done.

Keeping your excess weight shifted starts with two things: understanding how you became overweight in the first place, and identifying your motivation for wanting to change. Anyone who has already reached their goal weight should be able to identify their motivation very easily. They may even be able to identify their previous poor eating choices because they will presumably have overcome them — maybe only on a temporary basis — in order to achieve their current weight loss.

If you've done both of these things and have also read the self-hypnosis sessions through from start to finish — reinforcing all the Positive Thoughts — you should have put the GMB toolkit in place on a subconscious level, ensuring you have the means to avoid all your previously poor food choices in the future.

'I spent literally thousands of pounds on various pills, potions, shakes, even liposuction, and never succeeded in losing the weight permanently. Now, with Martin and Marion's help, I'm more than 2 stone (12.7kg) lighter, much happier and fitter. I've given all my big clothes away!'
GMB CLIENT W. L.

GMB for Shorter-Term Weight Loss

So far we've been looking at how to deal with *long-term* weight issues: making sure you know how to shed weight safely while learning how never to gain it back again.

Of course, it's possible that you might not have a long-term weight problem, but a *short-term* reason for being sure you're going to lose that little bit of extra weight. Getting married is a classic example, as are occasions such as an exotic beach holiday or a school or college prom.

Well, never fear! GMB's approach is equally applicable in these cases because, although it's not a 'crash diet', *if followed accurately*, it will *guarantee* weight loss at the widely accepted safe rate of 1–2lb (0.45–0.90kg) per week. So a size 14 bride-to-be who wants to wear a size 12 or 10 wedding dress in a few months' time can be sure she'll reach her target. If she chooses to continue following the system afterwards, it's entirely up to her. The ideal is to eat healthily, of course, so if any changes made for a short-term loss lead to a better level of nutrition – less fat, more fibre, more water – only good can come of it.

From Session 1 you can start the change, and, although you're likely to alter your relationship with food and food choices generally every bit as much as someone coming to the book with a high BMI and a considerable amount of weight to shift, you'll have a relatively shorter journey to reach your target.

There are other groups of people who could benefit from GMB's approach, including those with chronic illnesses or debilitating conditions either caused by, or made worse by, excess weight. Diabetics are perhaps the most obvious group. If you are diabetic, changing your eating habits is one of the first things your doctor will advise, and in the case of Type 2 diabetes there are indications that you can improve, or arguably completely eradicate, the condition, by losing weight through a healthier diet coupled with more exercise. Kay Lindley's experience in Chapter 10 supports this.

'I'd thought being overweight was due to one reason, but it soon became clear that it was a completely different thing! In 48 hours I've gone from stuffing my face (as a rebellious Type 2 diabetic) to – without even thinking about it – eating slowly and having only a quarter of the portion size I used to eat.'
GMB client **S.H.**

GMB for Young People

The number of obese children and teenagers is soaring; not far short of a million youngsters in the UK – about 30 per cent of 2–15 year olds – were classed as overweight or obese in 2010.[1]

In fact, researchers have predicted that in the near future a generation of parents will start to outlive their children because of the obesity-related problems their offspring will begin to suffer. Leading nutritionist Professor Andrew Prentice, from the London School of Hygiene and Tropical Medicine, estimates that being clinically obese shortens lifespan by some nine years. He describes the mix of obesity and a more sedentary lifestyle (25 per cent of British youngsters watch four hours TV a day) as an explosive mix.[2]

In 2005 the World Health Organization announced that, globally, there were 20 million overweight children under the age of five. In just five years this more than doubled to 42 million.[3] The International Obesity Task Force calculates that up to 200 million school-age children worldwide are overweight, and as many as 50 million of these are obese.[4] No longer regarded as 'puppy fat', overweight in childhood is now regarded as a strong indicator of obesity as an adult – and we've already looked at what that can lead to.

Obesity-related health problems in teenagers are similar to those seen in adults. However, the numbers are frighteningly large – more than 45 per cent of teens in the USA are at risk of developing illness and disease due to their weight,[5] and obese youngsters are 35 per cent more likely to die of cancer as adults.[6]

With some experts in the UK now saying that gastric balloons should be offered to children as young as 11,[7] perhaps it's time to educate these youngsters about only eating when they're hungry. Particularly given that the UK government's 2009 Change4Life programme suggested that 90 per cent of British youngsters will be overweight or obese by 2050 unless there's a radical change in eating habits and activity levels.[8] (In these times of recession, let's not forget that obesity is reckoned to cost the British economy more than £2 billion annually).[9] It's clear that the change needs to start now.

GMB is as relevant for young people as for anyone else. There's no dangerous fad, no food groups to cut out, no coding, points, or bans – just a way of recognizing how to alter your view of food, and what and when to eat.

In today's high-speed, high-tech society, the members of a household often don't share mealtimes and you can find all sorts of psychological implications from that apart from dietary ones. But fast food – if that's the choice of the teenager, or the schoolchild in a rush – is generally high-fat, low-nutrient, high-sugar, quick-fix stuff. It's the classic 'beige food' which anyone conscious of their weight and health should avoid in favour of fresh fruit and vegetables and other unprocessed foods.

Young people are also capable of understanding the blindingly obvious: if you eat more than your body needs, you'll get fat. And if you're fat you usually won't be as healthy as if you're slim; and if you're fat you won't be able to buy clothes as easily; and buying size 16 or 18 or 20 clothes won't be nearly as much fun as grabbing a standard size 12 from the rail, and so on and so forth.

The youngsters themselves may not be thinking long term, or even thinking of their health at all, but parents be aware: Type 2 diabetes, which is closely related to obesity, could knock 10 years off your kids' lives.[10] It's usually diagnosed in the over-40s but rates in children are rising rapidly.[11]

Perhaps the first step in ensuring young people eat a healthier diet, and address any weight problems they may be developing, would be to teach them to cook. If they can make themselves a tasty nutritious meal, and enjoy the process as well as eating the results, they'll have less need for junk food!

Teenagers experience bodily changes that are hard to live with, even if weight isn't an issue. Girls' hips broaden, and their breasts develop. They may feel that they don't compare to the girls they see on TV, and in magazines – especially if they haven't taken on board the significance of airbrushing in the perfection of those images. Guys develop at different rates, and washboard abs are usually found only on models in their 20s.

Teenagers who find it hard to control how much they eat may decide to follow an extreme diet. Often, though, this is followed by eating huge quantities of food, and, because they then feel guilty about their binge, they might make themselves vomit or take laxatives. Eating too little to remain at a healthy weight (anorexia), and eating followed by throwing up all the food (calories) they've eaten (bulimia) are both harmful eating disorders, and if you recognize these symptoms in yourself, or anyone you know, please see a doctor.

Weight Loss Tips for Teenagers:

- Take more exercise – just a bit every day to start with.

- Choose more fruit and vegetables, and cut out junk food and sauces.

- Cut out or cut down on sugary and carbonated drinks.

- Drink more water.

- Get on a bike!

- Cut out chips — remember they are higher in calories than plain boiled potatoes.

- Switch from white to wholemeal bread.

- Have smaller portion sizes and avoid second helpings.

- Avoid skipping meals, particularly breakfast.

What if I Hit a Plateau?

Everyone will have a plateau — maybe more than one — when shedding excess weight; these are, of course, nothing more than temporary blips, lapses that you pick yourself up from and move on. There might come a time, though, when some crisis occurs — perhaps the death of a loved one, emotional trauma, financial meltdown — which would understandably knock your focus totally away from the time and effort you've put into dealing with your food issues.

At the time you'll almost certainly think there's no getting back on track. You may even have no interest in getting back on track; you won't feel remotely inclined to even *think* about turning a corner, never mind doing it. In fact, although they are traumatic and upsetting, with regard to weight loss these occasions are actually no different from a plateau. They may feel worse, and be emotionally worse, but all you need to do is start afresh. Read the book from scratch. You haven't relapsed, you've had a lapse — and you *can* get over it.

A lot of people fear failure so much — and they really build it up. But there's nothing wrong with failure. We all fail at something some of the time. Just prepare for it and learn from it. After all, nobody can be perfect all of the time.

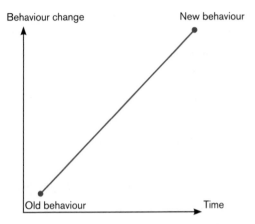

Successful behaviour change is rarely a smooth process

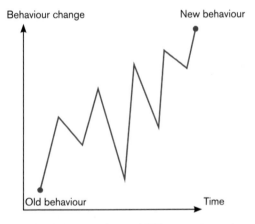

Each setback is only a lapse, NOT a complete relapse.

What if you're trying to shift some excess weight and you have a little lapse while on holiday? That's okay: you can put it right afterwards.

Don't fear failure – it doesn't have to be forever. Past failures have zero effect on future success.

WHAT YOU'VE LEARNED IN THIS CHAPTER
· ·

- If you've shed excess weight already, be sure to keep it off.

- The Gastric Mind Band can be used for both short- and long-term weight loss.

- Teenagers will be quite safe using our methods too.

- It doesn't matter how many times you start.

A Final Word

You've reached this point with our help – and maybe with support from your family and friends. From here on in, though, you'll most probably be relying on your own resources, and what you've learned from this book. Whenever you need us, we'll still be here – all the little stories, reminders, anecdotes, examples, proverbs... all the ammunition you need against the Diet Terrorists and others will still be right here within these pages.

Before you consign us to the bookshelf, though (only to be dusted down when you next have a bad day or a stressful week!), here's a reminder of the key GMB points to keep at the back (or front!) of your mind for when you face food choices – which, after all, is likely to be at least twice a day.

When you are eating something, remember the following:

- Ask yourself *why* you are eating it. If you are not hungry you don't need to eat.

- Take the word *want* out of your vocabulary and replace it with *need*. Try it...

- Might you be *thirsty*? Don't forget that some of the sensations of thirst are the same as for hunger. If you think you're hungry, drink some water, and don't eat unless you still feel hungry 10 minutes later.

- Are you eating *slowly* enough for your brain to have time to let you know when you're no longer hungry?

- Are you *tasting* the food and truly enjoying the flavour of it?

- Recall your *reasons* for wanting to become a healthy weight. What's more important – the quick fix or the longer-term goal and a healthier future life?

- You can always picture your *fork in the road* – where will you be and what will you feel like next month, or next year?

- Use your *Pause Button*. It can make all the difference if you just use it to put your thoughts on hold and give yourself time to reconsider the choice you're about to make.

The Future of GMB

Whatever happens with the expansion of the GMB brand, our own immediate plans are to continue offering the GMB treatment in person at our clinic in Fuengirola in southern Spain. We know that through meeting clients, providing therapy face to face, and working with their feedback, we're guaranteed to stay at the 'sharp end' of the treatment process, and are in the best position to improve and develop the GMB treatment. We believe that GMB has a significant part to play in the lives of the people we treat, and in the global battle against obesity.

Our first clinic grew to cater for our growing client list, and is now in a spacious top-floor suite almost (but not quite) overlooking the Mediterranean. Not a bad place to meet clients! GMB treatment may be the best known of our therapies, but it is only one of many others we offer, from Stop Smoking to relationship counselling.

Appendix

Height Conversion Chart

Feet/ inches	Metres/ cm	Feet/ inches	Metres/ cm	Feet/ inches	Metres/ cm
4ft 6in	1.37m	5ft 1in	1.55m	5ft 8in	1.73m
4ft 7in	1.39m	5ft 2in	1.57m	5ft 9in	1.75m
4ft 8in	1.42m	5ft 3in	1.60m	5ft 10in	1.78m
4ft 9in	1.45m	5ft 4in	1.63m	5ft 11in	1.80m
4ft 10in	1.47m	5ft 5in	1.65m	6ft 0in	1.83m
4ft 11in	1.50m	5ft 6in	1.68m	6ft 1in	1.85m
5ft 0in	1.52m	5ft 7in	1.70m	6ft 2in	1.88m

Weight Conversion Chart

Stones/ pounds	Pounds	Kilograms	Stones/ pounds	Pounds	Kilograms
9 0	126	57.2	10 9	149	67.6
9 1	127	57.6	10 10	150	68.0
9 2	128	58.1	10 11	151	68.5
9 3	129	58.5	10 12	152	68.9
9 4	130	59.0	10 13	153	69.4
9 5	131	59.4	11 0	154	69.9
9 6	132	59.9	11 1	155	70.3
9 7	133	60.3	11 2	156	70.8
9 8	134	60.8	11 3	157	71.2
9 9	135	61.2	11 4	158	71.7
9 10	136	61.7	11 5	159	72.1
9 11	137	62.1	11 6	160	72.6
9 12	138	62.6	11 7	161	73.0
9 13	139	63.0	11 8	162	73.5
10 0	140	63.5	11 9	163	73.9
10 1	141	64.0	11 10	164	74.4
10 2	142	64.4	11 11	165	74.8
10 3	143	64.9	11 12	166	75.3
10 4	144	65.3	11 13	167	75.7
10 5	145	65.8	12 0	168	76.2
10 6	146	66.2	12 1	169	76.7
10 7	147	66.7	12 2	170	77.1
10 8	148	67.1	12 3	171	77.6

Stones/ pounds	Pounds	Kilograms	Stones/ pounds	Pounds	Kilograms
12 4	172	78.0	14 0	196	88.9
12 5	173	78.5	14 1	197	89.4
12 6	174	78.9	14 2	198	89.8
12 7	175	79.4	14 3	199	90.3
12 8	176	79.8	14 4	200	90.7
12 9	177	80.3	14 5	201	91.2
12 10	178	80.7	14 6	202	91.6
12 11	179	81.2	14 7	203	92.1
12 12	180	81.6	14 8	204	92.5
12 13	181	82.1	14 9	205	93.0
13 0	182	82.6	14 10	206	93.4
13 1	183	83.0	14 11	207	93.9
13 2	184	83.5	14 12	208	94.3
13 3	185	83.9	14 13	209	94.8
13 4	186	84.4	15 0	210	95.3
13 5	187	84.8	15 1	211	95.7
13 6	188	85.3	15 2	212	96.2
13 7	189	85.7	15 3	213	96.6
13 8	190	86.2	15 4	214	97.1
13 9	191	86.6	15 5	215	97.5
13 10	192	87.1	15 6	216	98.0
13 11	193	87.5	15 7	217	98.4
13 12	194	88.0	15 8	218	98.9
13 13	195	88.4	15 9	219	99.3

Stones/ pounds	Pounds	Kilograms	Stones/ pounds	Pounds	Kilograms
15 10	220	99.8	17 6	244	110.7
15 11	221	100.2	17 7	245	111.1
15 12	222	100.7	17 8	246	111.6
15 13	223	101.2	17 9	247	112.0
16 0	224	101.6	17 10	248	112.5
16 1	225	102.1	17 11	249	112.9
16 2	226	102.5	17 12	250	113.4
16 3	227	103.0	17 13	251	113.9
16 4	228	103.4	18 0	252	114.3
16 5	229	103.9	18 1	253	114.8
16 6	230	104.3	18 2	254	115.2
16 7	231	104.8	18 3	255	115.7
16 8	232	105.2	18 4	256	116.1
16 9	233	105.7	18 5	257	116.6
16 10	234	106.1	18 6	258	117.0
16 11	235	106.6	18 7	259	117.5
16 12	236	107.0	18 8	260	117.9
16 13	237	107.5	18 9	261	118.4
17 0	238	109.3	18 10	262	118.8
17 1	239	109.8	18 11	263	119.3
17 2	240	108.9	18 12	264	119.7
17 3	241	109.3	18 13	265	120.2
17 4	242	109.8	19 0	266	120.7
17 5	243	110.2	19 1	267	121.1

Stones/ pounds	Pounds	Kilograms	Stones/ pounds	Pounds	Kilograms
19 2	268	121.6	20 12	292	132.5
19 3	269	122.0	20 13	293	132.9
19 4	270	122.5	21 0	294	133.4
19 5	271	122.9	21 1	295	133.8
19 6	272	123.4	21 2	296	134.3
19 7	273	123.8	21 3	297	134.7
19 8	274	124.3	21 4	298	135.2
19 9	275	124.7	21 5	299	135.6
19 10	276	125.2	21 6	300	136.1
19 11	277	125.6	21 7	301	136.5
19 12	278	126.1	21 8	302	137.0
19 13	279	126.6	21 9	303	137.4
20 0	280	127.0	21 10	304	137.9
20 1	281	127.5	21 11	305	138.3
20 2	282	127.9	21 12	306	138.8
20 3	283	128.4	21 13	307	139.3
20 4	284	128.8	22 0	308	139.7
20 5	285	129.3	22 1	309	140.2
20 6	286	129.7	22 2	310	140.6
20 7	287	130.2	22 3	311	141.1
20 8	288	130.6	22 4	312	141.5
20 9	289	131.1	22 5	313	142.0
20 10	290	131.5	22 6	314	142.4
20 11	291	132.0	22 7	315	142.9

Stones/ pounds	Pounds	Kilograms	Stones/ pounds	Pounds	Kilograms
22 8	316	143.3	24 4	340	154.2
22 9	317	143.8	24 5	341	154.7
22 10	318	144.2	24 6	342	155.1
22 11	319	144.7	24 7	343	155.6
22 12	320	145.2	24 8	344	156.0
22 13	321	145.6	24 9	345	156.5
23 0	322	146.1	24 10	346	156.9
23 1	323	146.5	24 11	346	157.4
23 2	324	147.0	24 12	348	157.9
23 3	325	147.4	24 13	349	158.3
23 4	326	147.9	25 0	350	158.8
23 5	327	148.3	25 1	351	159.2
23 6	328	148.8	25 2	352	159.7
23 7	329	149.2	25 3	353	160.1
23 8	330	149.7	25 4	354	160.5
23 9	331	150.1	25 5	355	161.0
23 10	332	150.6	25 6	356	161.5
23 11	333	151.0	25 7	357	162.0
23 12	334	151.5	25 8	358	162.3
23 13	335	152.0	25 9	359	163.0
24 0	336	152.4	25 10	360	163.2
24 1	337	152.9	25 11	361	164.0
24 2	338	153.3	25 12	362	164.2
24 3	339	153.8	25 13	363	164.6

Body Mass Index (BMI) Classification

Developed in the 19th century by Belgian statistician Adolphe Quetelet, BMI is a way of seeing whether a person's weight is appropriate for their height. It is usually calculated by dividing their weight in kilograms by the square of their height in metres (kg/m^2).

For example, if you weigh 70kg and are 1.75m tall, your BMI will be 22.9.

$70kg / (1.75\ m^2) = 70 / 3.06 = 22.9$

The table below shows the International Classification of adult underweight, overweight and obesity according to BMI:[1]

Classification	BMI (kg/m^2)	
	Principal cut-off points	Additional cut-off points
Underweight	<18.50	<18.50
Severe thinness	<16.00	<16.00
Moderate thinness	16.00–16.99	16.00–16.99
Mild thinness	17.00–18.49	17.00–18.49
Normal range	18.50–24.99	18.50–22.99
		23.00–24.99
Overweight	≥25.00	≥25.00
Pre-obese	25.00–29.99	25.00–27.49
		27.50–29.99
Obese	≥30.00	≥30.00
Obese class I	30.00–34.99	30.00–32.49
		32.50–34.99
Obese class II	35.00–39.99	35.00–37.49
		37.50–39.99
Obese class III	≥40.00	≥40.00

Here's a simplified version:

BMI (kg/m²)	Classification
18.5–24.9	Normal range
25–29.9	Overweight
30–40	Obese
40–49.9	Morbidly Obese
50+	Super Morbidly Obese

A report published at the end of 2010 showed that of nearly 1.5 million adults, those within 'normal' BMI ranges were at the lowest risk of death.[2]

. . . .

Further Resources

The Time Paradox, Philip Zimbardo and John Boyd, (Rider, 2010)
Pause Button Therapy, Martin Shirran, Marion Shirran, Fiona Graham (Hay House UK, 2012)
Hope with Eating Disorders, Lynn Crilly (Hay House, 2012)
The Beck Diet Solution, Judith Beck (Robinson, 2008)

Accredited GMB Providers

Clients visiting accredited GMB therapists can relax in the knowledge that each therapist has undertaken exclusive training with Martin and Marion Shirran, enabling them to provide bespoke GMB therapy packages. Certification will be visible at all centres.

Additionally, it is a requirement of accreditation that all therapists are aware of, and incorporate, the latest developments and improvements in GMB therapy, resulting from the permanently ongoing research being undertaken.

At the time of going to print, treatment centres were located in:

- Nicosia
- Seattle
- London
- Denmark

- Bahrain
- Dubai
- Abu Dhabi
- Malaga

To obtain up-to-date contact details and information regarding accredited GMB therapists and clinics, visit www.gmband.com

References

About this Book

1. http://www.asirt.org/KnowBeforeYouGo/RoadSafetyFacts/RoadCrashStatistics/tabid/13/Default.aspx
2. http://www.bbc.co.uk/health/physical_health/conditions/obesity.shtml

Chapter 1: Obese? Moi?

1. http://www.dailymail.co.uk/news/article-4984082.
2. http://win.niddk.nih.gov/publications/PDFs/stat904z.pdf
3. http://www.who.int/mediacentre/factsheets/fs311/en/
4. http://www.who.int/mediacentre/factsheets/fs311/en/
5. http://www.ic.nhs.uk/pubs/opad12
6. http://webarchive.nationalarchives.gov.uk/+/www.dh.gov.uk/en/Publichealth/Obesity/DH_078098
7. http://www.nhs.uk/news/2011/08August/Pages/half-of-uk-predicted-to-be-obese-by-2030.aspx
8. http://www.nelm.nhs.uk/en/NeLM-Area/News/2012---February/24/Report-says-weight-loss-stomach-surgery-up-12-per-cent-in-a-year-but-prescriptions-for-obesity-drugs-fall/
9. http://www.cancer.org/Cancer/CancerCauses/DietandPhysicalActivity/BodyWeightandCancerRisk/body-weight-and-cancer-risk-effects
10. http://media.wiley.com/product_data/excerpt/15/04700191/0470019115.pdf

11. http://win.niddk.nih.gov/publications/health_risks.htm
12. http://www.usatoday.com/news/health/medical/health/medical/
    diabetes/story/2011-11-13/Report-522M-people-could-have-
    diabetes-by-2030/51189950/1
13. http://www.guardian.co.uk/society/2012/apr/25/diabetes-
    treatment-bankrupt-nhs-generation
14. http://www.dailymail.co.uk/health/article-104806/How-Botox-
    help-stroke-victims.html http://www.stroke.org.uk/media_centre/
    facts_and_figures/index.html
15. http://info.cancerresearchuk.org/news/archive/pressrelease/
    2012-03-30-obesity-drives-kidney-cancer-cases-to-record-high
16. http://www.cancer.gov/cancertopics/factsheet/Risk/obesity
17. http://www.usatoday.com/news/health/medical/health/medical/
    heartdisease/story/2011/02/Obesity-alone-raises-risk-of-fatal-
    heart-attack-study-finds/43812248/1

Chapter 2: Giraffes, Sparrows and Obesity

1. http://archives.drugabuse.gov/TXManuals/CBT/CBT11.html
2. http://en.wikipedia.org/wiki/Low_frustration_tolerance
3. http://www.dailymail.co.uk/health/article-2117445/
4. http://news.sky.com/home/article/1248595
5. http://en.wikipedia.org/wiki/Lateral_hypothalamus
6. http://blogs.plos.org/obesitypanacea/2011/05/13/the-science-of-
   starvation-how-long-can-humans-survive-without-food-or-water/
7. http://www.dummies.com/how-to/content/how-your-brain-signals-
   your-bodys-need-for-food.html
8. http://www.pureandhealthy.com/blog/2010/08/hungry-you-could-
   be-confusing-it-for-thirst/
9. http://www.csun.edu/~vcpsy00h/students/hunger.htm

Chapter 3: Anyone for Gastric Band Surgery?

1. http://www.dailymail.co.uk/home/you/article-2124641/The-skinny-
   Weight-loss-surgery.html
   http://www.bupa.co.uk/individuals/health-information/directory/g/
   gastric-band#textBlock223474
2. http://www.bospa.org/Information
3. http://www.nbt.nhs.uk/our-services/a-z-services/bariatric-surgery/
   bariatric-operations
4. http://www.ncbi.nlm.nih.gov/pubmed/18387472

5. http://www.logicalmetrics.com/news/consumer-product-quality-assurance-news/media-industry-blogs-and-news-sources/consumer-union/consumer-reports/c2408c988f0003a057f6cdfc2b1ea062
6. http://www.dailymail.co.uk/health/article-1292350/From-brittle-bones-depression-suicide-true-costs-gastric-bands--watch-Vanessa-Feltz--lose-weight.html
7. http://www.bospa.org/Information

Chapter 5: The Sessions: A Life-Changing Sequence

1. http://www.korr.com/products/metacheck-info.html

Chapter 6: Session 1: Peeling the Onion

1. http://www.health.harvard.edu/blog/why-eating-slowly-may-help-you-feel-full-faster-20101019605
2. http://www.drcederquist.com/weight-loss-library/physicians-weight-loss.aspx/Do-artificial-sweetners-make-you-eat-more.aspx
3. http://en.wikipedia.org/wiki/Transtheoretical_model
   http://www.doi.vic.gov.au/doi/doielect.nsf/2a6bd98dee287482ca256915001cff0c/eac8a984b717095bca256d100017ba50/$FILE/Theories and models behaviour change.pdf
4. http://www.womentowomen.com/insulinresistance/default.aspx
5. http://www.rodale.com/michael-pollan
6. http://www.dailymail.co.uk/health/article-1256509/Eating-fruit-make-fat.html
7. http://www.metabolicprecision.com/articles-1/alcohol-increases-appetite
8. http://www.hornetjuice.com/how-long-does-alcohol-affect-your-fat-burning-metabolism.html
9. http://en.wikipedia.org/wiki/Low_frustration_tolerance
10. http://www.agendamag.com/content/2011/01/did-you-know-sugar-makes-you-eat-more-offsets-your-mood-and-ruins-your-looks/
11. http://www.dailymail.co.uk/femail/article-1358557/
12. http://www.bmi-calculator.net/waist-to-hip-ratio-calculator/waist-to-hip-ratio-chart.php

Chapter 8: Session 2: Understanding What Your Body Needs

1. http://exercise.about.com/cs/fitnesstools/g/BMR.htm
2. http://www.best-ab-workout.com/resting-metabolic-rate-rmr/

3. http://www.shapesense.com/nutrition/articles/thermic-effect-of-food.aspx
4. http://www.sharecare.com/question/thermic-effect-activity
5. http://dukechronicle.com/article/scientists-find-possible-genetic-link-obesity
6. http://www.bariatric-surgery-source.com/causes-of-obesity.html
7. http://www.ideafit.com/fitness-library/keeping-hunger-bay
8. http://voices.yahoo.com/refined-foods-may-lead-addiction-6435542.html
9. http://www.dailymail.co.uk/news/article-1170783/
10. http://www.nhs.uk/Livewell/loseweight/Pages/10000stepschallenge.aspx
11. http://www.medindia.net/news/Protein-Rich-Breakfast-Successfully-Wards-Off-Hunger-Pangs-85306-1.htm
12. http://forecast.diabetes.org/magazine/food-thought/eating-colorful-food-has-health-benefits
13. http://www.freedrinkingwater.com/water-education/water-senior.htm
14. http://www.livestrong.com/article/441564-difference-between-being-hungry-and-thirsty/
15. http://www.saga.co.uk/health/healthy-eating/how-much-water-do-we-need.aspx
16. http://www.h2oasispurewater.com/Water_Facts.html
17. http://www.betterhealth.vic.gov.au/bhcv2/bhcarticles.nsf/pages/water_a_vital_nutrient?open
18. http://www.benefits-of-honey.com/how-much-water-should-you-drink-a-day.html
19. http://www.phlaunt.com/lowcarb/19058097.php
20. http://www.telegraph.co.uk/science/science-news/3296662/When-DID-we-start-getting-fat.html
21. http://www.neoseeker.com/forums/18/t1228954-ways-to-burn-off-big-mac/
22. http://www.livestrong.com/article/368575-why-does-metabolism-slow-with-age/
23. http://www.nutracheck.co.uk/Library/WeightLoss/which-weighs-more-fat-or-muscle_1.html
24. http://www.telegraph.co.uk/science/science-news/8514093/Eating-in-front-of-television-leads-to-snacking.html
25. http://tinyurl.com/8jv7emk
26. http://auto.howstuffworks.com/question527.htm

Chapter 10: Session 3: Weight Loss in Five Words

1. http://www.motivationalinterview.net/clinical/motmodel.htm
2. http://library.thinkquest.org/3750/taste/taste.html
3. http://www.spring.org.uk/2009/09/how-long-to-form-a-habit.php
4. http://tinyurl.com/7vl7n5s
5. p.29 *The Beck Diet Solution,* Robinson (2007)

Chapter 12: Session 4: The Gastric Mind Band

1. http://www.mamashealth.com/organs/stomach.asp
2. http://www.ajronline.org/content/186/2/522.full
   http://www.crospon.com/bariatrictimes.pdf
3. http://hypertextbook.com/facts/2000/JonathanCheng.shtml
4. ttp://www.ajronline.org/content/189/3/681.full
5. http://www.bospa.org/Information
   http://www.gastricband.org.uk/gastric-band-success-rates.html
6. http://www.medpagetoday.com/MeetingCoverage/ASMBS/20919
7. http://www.bospa.org/Information

Chapter 14: A Reminder of the Health Risks of Obesity

1. http://www.nhs.uk/Conditions/Diabetes-type2/Pages/Introduction.aspx
2. http://digestive.niddk.nih.gov/ddiseases/pubs/gallstones/
3. http://osteoarthritis.about.com/od/osteoarthritis101/a/obesity.htm
4. http://www.telegraph.co.uk/health/healthnews/4937256/Obesity-increases-the-likelihood-of-knee-replacement-research-shows.html
5. http://www.heart.org/HEARTORG/GettingHealthy/WeightManagement/Obesity/Obesity-Information_UCM_307908_Article.jsp
6. http://tinyurl.com/82subf8
7. http://obesity.ygoy.com/2009/03/16/obesity-a-major-risk-factor-for-gout/
8. http://www.spineuniverse.com/conditions/back-pain/back-pain-obesity
9. http://info.cancerresearchuk.org/healthyliving/obesityandweight /howdoweknow/body-weight-and-cancer-the-evidence
10. www.nhs.uk/cancer
11. http://www.guardian.co.uk/science/2007/dec/11/medicalresearch.health

12. http://coloncancer.about.com/od/stagesandsurvivalrate1/a/ColonCancerSurv.htm
13. http://tinyurl.com/93smwrx
14. http://www.mydr.com.au/asthma/obesity-and-asthma
15. http://bupa.co.uk/individuals/health-information/directory/s/hi-snoring
16. http://www.medicinenet.com/script/main/art.asp?articlekey=46582
17. http://archpsyc.jamanetwork.com/article.aspx?articleid=210608
18. http://tinyurl.com/9tfurud;
    http://tinyurl.com/8ao2cje
19. http://vitals.msnbc.msn.com/_news/2012/03/13/10674252-obese-men-at-greater-risk-for-infertility?lite
20. http://www.sciencedaily.com releases/2010/10/ 101010133620.htm

Chapter 15: Your GMB Journey Continues

1. http://www.ic.nhs.uk/pubs/opad12
2. http://www.dailymail.co.uk/news/article-137440/
3. http://www.who.int/dietphysicalactivity/childhood/en/
4. http://www.iaso.org/iotf/obesity/obesitytheglobalepidemic/
5. http://www.teenhelp.com/teen-health/teen-obesity.html
6. http://www.dailymail.co.uk/health/article-2004039/
7. http://www.dailymail.co.uk/health/article-2052581/Obese-children-young-11-gastric-implant-NHS.html
8. http://www.getsurrey.co.uk/news/s/2043559 _vision_of_obesity_highlights_change4life_campaign
9. http://www.bupa.co.uk/business/employer-health-hub/general-health-fitness/obesity-business-issue
10. http://www.diabetes.co.uk/diabetes-life-expectancy.html
11. http://www.telegraph.co.uk/health/healthnews/5394255/Cases-of-diabetes-in-children-will-increase-70-per-cent-by-2020.html

Appendix

1. http://apps.who.int/bmi/index.jsp?introPage=intro_3.html World Health Organization Global Database on Body Mass Index
2. http://blogs.scientificamerican.com/observations/2010/12/01/the-best-body-mass-indexes-for-low-mortality-rates/

Index

The abbreviations GMB, NLP and PBT stand for Gastric Mind Band, Neuro-Linguistic Programming and Pause Button Therapy respectively.

Pause Button Therapy

Martin and Marion Shirran

with Fiona Graham

How helpful would it be if we could occasionally just pause, freeze time for a few moments and consider the consequences of the actions are about to take?

Pause Button Therapy® is a proven, innovative and interactive therapy technique that allows you to do exactly this, empowering you to break free of negative habits and unconscious responses. PBT is based on an incredibly simple idea but can be used for a whole host of issues. It provides additional thinking time, allowing a person to consider the potential outcomes of their actions and adjust their behaviour accordingly.

PBT has been hugely successful in the treatment of everything from addictions and weight issues to depression, anxiety and relationship problems, and this book will show you the many ways in which you can use it to transform your experience of life.

'PBT is wonderfully simple, but simply effective.'
Stelios N. Georgiou, Professor of Educational Psychology, University of Cyprus

'I know that this book will be treasured by many readers from all backgrounds.'
Professor Philip G. Zimbardo, San Francisco, USA

Published by Hay House

JOIN THE HAY HOUSE FAMILY

As the leading self-help, mind, body and spirit publisher in the UK, we'd like to welcome you to our family so that you can enjoy all the benefits our website has to offer.

 EXTRACTS from a selection of your favourite author titles

 COMPETITIONS, PRIZES & SPECIAL OFFERS Win extracts, money off, downloads and so much more

 LISTEN to a range of radio interviews and our latest audio publications

 CELEBRATE YOUR BIRTHDAY An inspiring gift will be sent your way

 LATEST NEWS Keep up with the latest news from and about our authors

 ATTEND OUR AUTHOR EVENTS Be the first to hear about our author events

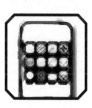 **iPHONE APPS** Download your favourite app for your iPhone

 HAY HOUSE INFORMATION Ask us anything, all enquiries answered

Join us online at **www.hayhouse.co.uk**

 292B Kensal Road, London W10 5BE
T: 020 8962 1230 E: info@hayhouse.co.uk

ABOUT THE AUTHORS

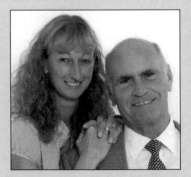

Martin and Marion Shirran undertook a diploma course in Clinical Hypnotherapy together before moving from the UK to Spain, where in 2004 they established the Elite Clinics to put into practice their shared love of helping people. Their Gastric Mind Band© weight-loss therapy is now widely emulated by other clinics and therapists. Martin sees it as a case of imitation being the sincerest form of flattery!

Intrigued by psychology since taking a course on sales and marketing, Martin undertook a Rational Emotive Behaviour Therapy (REBT) course at Birmingham University, NLP training and is a member of the International Hypnosis Research Institute. Marion holds an honours degree from Lancaster University. Both Martin and Marion hold diplomas in Clinical Hypnosis and are certified and registered with the American Board of Hypnotherapy and the British Institute of Hypnotherapy. They are also independently registered with the Complementary and Natural Healthcare Council in the UK. Marion and Martin read widely on psychology, and have become prolific writers on the subject of their therapy and hypnosis.

In their spare time, Martin enjoys flying and sailing while Marion's number-one pastime is cooking. The pair sees GMB as an ongoing project that they're happy to revise with the experience of every new client. Finding new insights and solutions is something they not only do, but revel in.

Fiona Graham, formerly a journalist in the UK, worked with Marion and Martin on their first book for Hay House, *Pause Button Therapy*, and was more than happy to step up for this, their second publication.

www.gmband.com